PLAIN TALK
ABOUT
ACUPUNCTURE

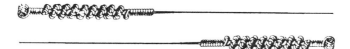

Ellinor R. Mitchell

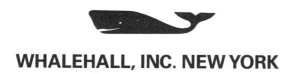

WHALEHALL, INC. NEW YORK

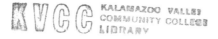

Mitchell, Ellinor R.
  Plain Talk About Acupuncture

ISBN 0-9617918-0-2

Cover, Book Design, and Illustrations: Ray Gordon

Manufactured in the United States of America by The Studley
Press, Inc., Dalton, MA 01226.

WHALEHALL, INC.
277 West End Avenue, # 15 A, New York, NY 10023

To Ray Gordon
with love and admiration

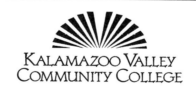

CONTENTS

FOREWORD

The lucky readers of this book have access to a wonderful storehouse of information about acupuncture. Many practitioners (myself included) have been waiting somewhat impatiently for this publication. Our patients ask, "What can I read?" and until this moment there was really no single book to give them. Now we have one.

Plain Talk About Acupuncture is a wide-ranging, intelligently written and superbly researched book. It contains everything from common sense (plain talk), to explanations of such things as endorphins and placebo effect, to the latest on veterinary acupuncture. Every page is full of the author's fascination with the subject, and reveals her interest in the down-to-earth nature of acupuncture. There are many examples of patients' experiences that give a real-life view of the kinds of conditions that can be treated, and what can be expected from acupuncture treatment. Because this is a patients' "guidebook" there is a large proportion of practical case-oriented information—what a treatment feels like, how to find a reliable acupuncturist, and so on.

There is very little explanation of the theoretics of Traditional Chinese Medicine, and to my way of thinking, this is as it should be. There are many theoretical books available for those who are interested. Patients are generally looking for relief from their illnesses, and not for introductions to medical theory. They are also looking for detailed information that will help them find treatment, and that is what this book so wonderfully provides. I will be sending crowds of patients to storm the bookstores for this book the moment it comes out.

Martha Howard, MD, Dipl. AC. NCCA

FOREWORD

The substance abuse chapter of this book is uniquely valuable to our field. Ms. Mitchell has resisted the temptation to refer to substance abuse only in terms of symptom relief or stress relief. She emphasizes the need for counselling as well as acupuncture. Her discussion is oriented to the needs *and* the ambivalence that people feel when they consider seeking substance abuse treatment. Ms. Mitchell's chapter is written with great sensitivity concerning the critical issues people feel when beginning substance abuse treatment.

In recent years many acupuncurists have begun to work with substance abuse clients and programs. Acupuncture has been an excellent benefit to this field, but only for those acupuncturists who have been well integrated with established substance abuse counselling and self-help modalities. Acupuncture develops the client's internal healing energy so that all phases of treatment are improved.

Michael O. Smith, M.D., D. Ac.
Division of Substance Abuse
Lincoln Hospital
Chairperson, National Acupuncture
Detoxification Association (NADA)

INTRODUCTION

Most writing about acupuncture is meant for medical scientists, health professionals, or students of Oriental medicine. As a physician, acupuncturist, and editor of medical publications, I know the complexities of writing about this subject. Colleagues share a background in science and technical language. But for non-professional readers, technical scientific language often obscures ideas. On the other hand, attempts to explain a difficult subject in ordinary language can be overly simplistic, and lead to misunderstanding. Too often, the prospective patient is either baffled or dissatisfied by currently available literature in this field.

Ellinor Mitchell tells about acupuncture like a very observant traveller talking to people who want to know if the trip is worthwhile. There is no doubt in my mind that Ms. Mitchell has made the journey: her information is accurate; and is presented in easily understandable language which demystifies acupuncture. Her book is practical, not theoretical.

One strength of the book is the author's ability to focus on the concerns and attitudes of people who wonder if they should try acupuncture treatment. This perspective is informed by a variety of anecdotal cases in which acupuncture patients speak of their treatment experiences.

Practicing acupuncturists quite properly devote time to

patient education. Of course there is no substitute for the practitioner's attentive response to a patient's questions. However, many people need the reinforcement of written material in order to remember what the acupuncturist told them. In this regard, Ms. Mitchell's book is extremely useful for any health professional's office.

Prospective patients, and those with a modest experience of acupuncture treatment, will find *Plain Talk About Acupuncture* reliable and enlightening. I also recommend this book highly to them, as well.

Jerome Wei-Ping Loh, MD, Ph.D,
FACP, FRCP, Lic.Ac. (NY)
Clinical Professor Emeritus,
State University of New York

ACKNOWLEDGEMENTS

This book has thrived "on the kindness of strangers."

Acupuncture patients made a major contribution to the book, which was conceived as an objective, practical guide for people who want to know what acupuncture can do for their health problems; what acupuncture treatment feels like; how to find a competent acupuncturist; and more.

It seemed logical to start by talking to people who had been treated with acupuncture. For objectivity's sake, I chose to look randomly for interviews. More than 30 patients spoke about their acupuncture treatment for musculoskeletal, systemic, and psychotherapeutic conditions. Each of them gave valuable information. Their generous participation enlivened research and encouraged me.

Another 98 patients responded to a newspaper notice. Letters came from all over the United States and from abroad— Bermuda, Holland, Japan, and Spain. Some people said acupuncture was useless. Some described musculoskeletal problems which, after years of resisting conventional treatment, yielded to acupuncture treatment. Others told of illness with no definable pathology, but powerfully depressing affect, which was finally alleviated by acupuncture treatment. Some people described inter-related physical, mental and emotional effects of their acupuncture treatment. Others saw their health problems as purely physical. A few letters moved me deeply by their modest gallantry. They may not see themselves in the book, but their vivid communications reinforced other research and enriched the material.

Acupuncturists trained in various traditions; physicians who know acupuncture and physicians who don't; public-health officials and other people concerned with acupuncture in the United States have given their time for interviews; and taken the trouble to write letters to this unknown inquirer. Others have opened doors for me to observe acupuncture classes, acupuncture treatment, special training sessions, and professional conferences.

With the understanding that their good offices in no way imply responsibility for the author's material, my thanks to: Dr. Robert H.O. Bannerman whose helpful comments on work-in-progress gave me confidence in continuing; Naida Colby, RN, for a memorable afternoon at the Sister Kenny Institute Pain Clinic in Minneapolis; Janis Cripe for cordial facilitation at the Second Conference of the Traditional Acupuncture Foundation, in Washington, DC; Dr. William David Graham, for illuminating discussions; Dr. Frederick F. Kao; Ginger McRae, Esq, whose brilliant *Critical Overview of U.S. Acupuncture Regulation* is a model of completeness and clarity; New York Society of Acupuncture for Physicians and Dentists; Martha Robinson who said, "What you need is a printout," and provided one; Dr. Allen M. Schoen who kindly permitted repeated observation of veterinary acupuncture; Dr. Mark Seem for visits to Tri-State Institute of Traditional Chinese Acupuncture; Sandra Stanton; and especially to Dr. Roger W.-M. Tsao for generous introductions, and for sustained encouragement of this project.

Friends and family have nourished this book. They balance the necessary equation, work and love.

Ellinor R. Mitchell
New York City and
Chilmark, Massachusetts

PREFACE

You may have heard about people in the United States having acupuncture treatment. Your niece in California says it helped a friend drop the twenty pounds she gained after her first child and couldn't lose in five years. A friend-of-friend was finally rid of incapacitating migraine headaches after a course of acupuncture treatment. Someone at the tennis court was told of another player whose tennis elbow was relieved by acupuncture. You've heard rumors of chronic ailments being helped by acupuncture—systemic lupus, ulcers, bronchial asthma, and many others. The problem with this good news is that none of it is firsthand. All that may *sound* well and good, but you want to know about acupuncture before you try it yourself. These are some of the questions most commonly asked by people considering acupuncture treatment.

- Is acupuncture safe?
- Acupuncture is so Chinese—does it work for non-Asians?

- Do you have to believe in acupuncture for it to work?
- Can acupuncture harm you? Should some people avoid it?
- Are there health problems for which acupuncture is definitely not recommended?
- What diseases may be treated by acupuncture?
- Is acupuncture expensive?
- Do they sterilize acupuncture needles?
- Does acupuncture hurt?
- How do you find a competent acupuncturist?
- Does health insurance cover acupuncture treatment?
- Do doctors approve of acupuncture?
- If acupuncture is real treatment, why don't more doctors recommend it?

Because acupuncture is not yet a standard treatment option for United States patients, you naturally want good reasons for considering this therapy. This book is for you. Along with answers to these questions and more, it includes patients' own stories of what it's like to experience acupuncture treatment, and the responses you can expect. It also contains useful resources, including a bibliography.

In an era of increasingly dehumanized health care, when the art and science of medicine is often reduced to the science alone, onset of a health problem can cause panic. Some people relieve this anxiety by unquestioning reliance on one medical authority. Others cope with fear by taking an active part in decisions about the care of their health.

To make sensible decisions, you need an informed choice of effective treatments. This book will help you judge if acupuncture can be useful to you, either as a first method of dealing with your health problem, or as a complement to standard medical practice.

ONE

Acupuncture in the United States

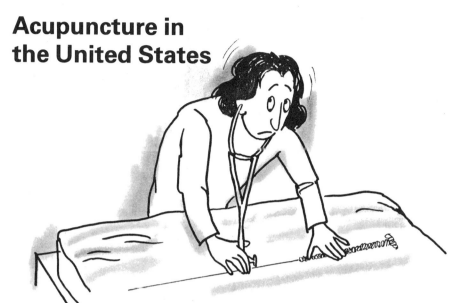

ACUPUNCTURE! Suddenly we read a lot about it in the early 1970s, when "table tennis diplomacy" was the catchword for reopening relations with China. While accompanying the U.S. Table Tennis team, James Reston of *The New York Times* came down with appendicitis. His account of effective needle-therapy for severe postoperative pain appeared in the *Times* in July, 1971; and prompted a nationwide surge of interest in this feature of Oriental Medicine.

It wasn't the first time in the history of East-West relations that fresh contact with China produced remarkable stories. In the popular press, journalists and doctors who had been to China, exposed us to a wide range of attitudes about acupuncture—from scornful disbelief to insistence that it was the greatest thing since sliced bread. The sensational phase of the acupuncture story ended after a few years. However, the early 1970s interest combined with other factors to spark a movement in the United States to establish acupuncture as an independent, generally accepted, well-regulated mode of health care. What are some of these other factors?

As always, the practice of acupuncture continued in United States Chinese communities. Most patients were of Asian origin, but the late 1960s saw an increase in non-Asians seeking treatment. A few of these people began to study acupuncture, here or abroad. Others told friends that acupuncture was effective drug-free treatment for many common problems. In different parts of the United States informal acupuncture networks developed, composed of practitioners and clients.

So long as it was confined to the Chinatowns of America, federal and state government never regulated the practice of acupuncture. Officially it was seen as just another ethnic cultural activity, like the celebration of Chinese New Year.

✳ ✳ ✳

American doctors who went to observe the organization and practice of medicine in China were intrigued by a technique iniatated there in 1958: the performance of major surgery using acupuncture analgesia instead of total anesthesia. The patients remained conscious. You may have seen pictures of patients talking to doctors and nurses during lung surgery. This might not be your cup of tea, but you probably know of the risks in general anesthesia, like lung collapse or blockage in a blood vessel of the lung. Also, without the trauma to the system caused by a period of total unconsciousness, patients recover more rapidly from the effects of surgery. Then, too, some operations can be better performed when the patient can cooperate with the surgeon. Observing serious operations on conscious, responsive patients made a striking impression on American doctors, even though, as one said, "I saw it but I didn't believe it!"

Outside general public attention medical journals reported news of Western scientific investigation of acupuncture. Medical scientists were not exploring virgin territory: acupuncture was introduced into the West in the 17th century. Interest in it has waxed and waned ever since, never completely dying out. Some United States doctors practiced and evaluated acupuncture in the early 19th century; among them was Benjamin Franklin's great-grandson, Dr. Franklin Bache, who translated into English one of seven contemporary French books on the subject.

Growth of scientific research in this field since 1971 sends a useful message to prospective acupuncture patients. Research depends on grants to pay for the work. Existence of a significant amount of research means that institutional funds are allocated to the subject. This shows some interest on the part of official science in taking acupuncture seriously, rather than dismissing it as irrelevant to health care in the West. Acupuncture is no medical hula hoop.

Early research goals emphasized application—what acupuncture was good for. Investigation of its usefulness in dentistry; and its effectiveness in treating sensori-neural deafness, paralysis, respiratory problems and chronic pain lead the field in the early 1970s. From 1975, emphasis was on figuring out how acupuncture works—what makes it tick. To date no complete scientific explanation has been established. It is difficult to fit acupuncture into the framework and vocabulary of Western science. However, biochemistry and clinical investigation have yielded some suggestions.

❊   ❊   ❊

Acupuncture is a system of healing, and of relieving pain, by sticking very fine solid needles into specific points on the body. Many acu-points are on or near nerves; their location suggests that needle therapy stimulates the central nervous system—the brain and spinal cord; and the autonomic nervous system—cells and fibers dealing with reflex actions. Acupuncture stimulates the body's capacity to resist or overcome ailments. In ways still not perfectly understood, acupuncture also prompts a biochemical response which decreases or eliminates painful sensations. Properly administered, this treatment produces no adverse effects.

Acupuncture originated in China, where it was practiced in early forms as long ago as 1,200 BC. By the 3rd century AD the fundamentals had been established and the system was nearly complete. Within the framework of Oriental medicine, which includes herbs, massage and exercise, Chinese doctors elaborated theories and applications of acupuncture during succeeding centuries; and the techniques became known outside China. In the 20th century changes in technique and application developed in China and other countries. In the continuous process of change, acupuncture adapts to different uses in different societies. Modern innovations include the use of low-voltage electro-acupuncture; laser acupuncture; and injection of Western medication at acupoints, which is said to lessen the amount of medication required for effective treatment. Modern applications include the use of acupuncture, often in conjunction with Lidocaine or Novocaine, for performance of major surgery without total anesthesia.

During the past decade clinical studies have shown that significant numbers of patients who had tried other remedies for profound recurrent pain of backache, headache, arthritis, sciatica and other incapacitating ailments, had good to excellent long-term relief after a series of acupuncture treatments. Patients quoted in this book—identified by the author, not from practitioners' clienteles—found acupuncture effective as treatment for various kinds of illness.

Barriers remain to acceptance of acupuncture by the American scientific establishment. Knowing the reasons for some official objections will equip you to weigh them against the realities of your own situation, and help you make an informed choice of treatment.

Acupuncture terms of description are alien to Western science. 16th century Chinese doctors used the term *ch'i* to describe energy that circulates through *meridians*. When the Englishman William Harvey published his description of the circulation of blood, in the 17th century, he inadvertently agreed with the Chinese in saying a fixed amount of blood circulates through the body; but Harvey didn't mention energy. The idea of energy moving through the body, or being blocked and causing imbalance which results in sickness, is basic to Oriental Medicine and acupuncture. But, as an American doctor said recently, "That is not the physiology we were taught."

Strenuous efforts to match acupuncture and Western medical concepts on a one-to-one basis generate more heat than light. Possibily *ch'i* is what Western science knows as the low-grade electrical current produced by the human body. One explanation of *meridians* is that early in the development of acupuncture Chinese doctors observed that stimulation of specific acu-points produced a particular response in patients with certain clusters of signs and symptoms. Grouping these points, and stimulating them in effective sequence, led to associating them in repeatable patterns. Possibly acu-points were codified into *meridians*—functions of various organs or groups of organs—the way we identify the North Star by reference to the Big Dipper.

Scholars say that interpreting centuries-old Chinese medical literature is tricky. All living languages change: think how Chaucer's 14th century English differs from our American language! Words themselves shift meaning over long periods of time. In English, 'girl' originally meant a youth of either sex. Chinese is no exception to this process of linguistic change.

To add to the confusion of medical historians, some terms describing theory and practice of acupuncture could have been used by innovative physicians to keep their methods secret. Competition among doctors for fame and money is neither a new practice nor limited to any one culture.

* * *

Some Western medical scientists say they distrust acupuncture because it is empirical medicine—developed from experience and observation, but not based on systematic theory or science. It is useful to remember that for over 70 years MDs used a particular medication empirically, without understanding its mechanism, just because it worked. Not until 1971 was a scientific explanation produced for how aspirin works to relieve pain.

We don't yet have satisfactory answers to the question of how acupuncture works. Its mechanism hasn't yet been completely analyzed, although biochemists, neurologists, pharmacologists and other scientists are closing in on the target. Some suggestions come from research designed specifically to examine acupuncture. In 1985 a French medical team demonstrated the movement of radioactive tracers along pathways which match classical Chinese

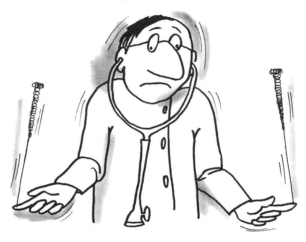

acupuncture meridians. Other insights have emerged from research aimed in different directions. In science as in life, exploration produces useful surprises: Columbus was looking for India, not North America.

Brain chemistry and cellular receptors became a hot topic of medical research in the mid-1970s. A chemical—made inside or outside the body—fits a specific receptor like a key in a lock. One kind of receptor locks onto opium. Researchers asked why—surely nature didn't provide us with opiate receptors just in case we got around to finding use for the opium poppy. Biochemical research led to identification of the body's self-produced pain-killers, endogenous morphine-like substances called *endorphins.* Clinical tests have shown that acupuncture stimulates endorphin release in both humans and animals.

One theory says that acupuncture stimulates nerve impulses to "plug the switchboard" through which pain messages go from an injury to the brain. 50% of known acu-points are connected to neural structures, 30% are near such structures, and 15% are not connected to nerves. This suggests that acupuncture stimulates the central nervous system—the brain and spinal cord; and the autonomic nervous system. The autonomic system regulates actions not controlled by our will, like those of the heart, lungs and intestine, and response of eye-pupils to light.

Eastern and Western medicine share the observation that the body's natural tendency is to heal itself, to restore *homeostasis,* a relatively stable internal environment. This idea underlies old as well as new western approaches to health care. There was even a Latin phrase to express it: *vis medicatrix naturae,* the healing power of nature. The drive to restore balance is a fundamental indicator of health. In Sweden a pioneer senior medical researcher has published a theory of biologically closed electrical circuits functioning as an additional circulatory system. One by-product of his work is a suggestion that bioelectrical processes acount for the mechanism of acupuncture.

Acupuncture has been shown to improve functioning of the immune system. The preventive aspect of acupuncture treatment lies in its ability to stimulate body processes to correct imbalances, and maintain the desired equilibrium. A recent study in Taiwan showed that white blood cells increase when a point on the hand is needled. To produce its normalizing effect, acupuncture works by insinuation, not by a frontal assault on disease.

It is interesting to note that two recent advances in Western medicine reflect these acupuncture principles of *balance* and *insinuation.* In 1982 the Nobel Prize in Medicine was given for research into *prostaglandins,* which nobody had ever heard of before the late 1930s. Hormone-like chemicals which are found in nearly every body cell, prostaglandins often work in opposing pairs. There seems to be a connection between some problems caused by injury, stress or disease, and prostaglandin imbalance. In 1984 the Nobel Prize in Medicine was given to immunologists for research which produced *monoclonal antibodies,* fused cells which can, at very fine levels of distinction, diagnose and undermine various categories of disease.

❋   ❋   ❋

Some people ask if doctors approve of acupuncture. Others, with no relief after many visits to doctors, don't care: pain and frustration make them despair of help from conventional medicine. If the question concerns you, here are some things to bear in mind when you evaluate a doctor's judgement of acupuncture.

The American Medical Association (AMA) defines acupuncture as "experimental treatment." Representing about 50% of practicing physicians in the United States, the AMA is a strong lobby for conservative official medicine, which changes policy slowly. The first revision of the AMA Code of Ethics in 25 years only recently removed injunctions against professional association with anyone practicing a non-scientific specialty. Exclusivity is a recurrent theme in medicine: French doctors in the 14th century refused to associate with surgeons, because surgeons worked with their hands. . .

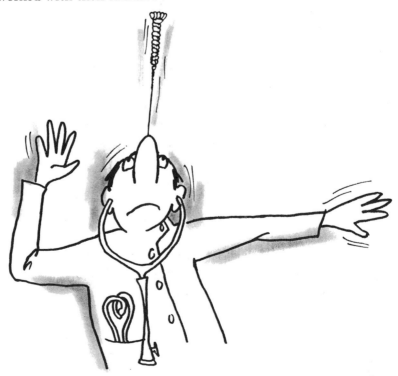

When the Food and Drug Administration (FDA) set guidelines for sales of acupuncture devices, it was strongly influenced by AMA policy, expressed by doctors who were unfamiliar with acupuncture. Insisting that the tools of acupuncture be labelled "experimental" was a bureaucratic way to call the treatment "experimental" as well.

Official medicine takes a possessive attitude toward acupuncture, wanting it kept under the supervision of doctors. For this purpose it might seem reasonable to teach acupuncture in medical schools, as is done in the Scandinavian countries. But acupuncture is not routinely taught in U.S. medical schools.

The AMA is a lobby; doctors are individuals. A few will recommend acupuncture to their patients as a first choice of treatment for some conditions. Others may suggest it as a last resort: doctors become frustrated when their treatment fails to help a patient. Some doctors still make patients feel foolish for even asking about acupuncture. However, many will say frankly that they don't know much about it, but from what they've heard, it might be worth a try. As one open-minded medical specialist said, "I'm for anything if it works." You might wonder, if acupuncture is real treatment, why doctors don't recommend it as a matter of course. Generally, because they don't know what acupuncture can do.

In the early 1970s some observers insisted that acupuncture was culture-specific—"It's so Chinese, how can it work for non-Asians?" people asked. "It works on Chinese because they are used to the idea," said a doctor who travels internationally as a medical consultant. More dismaying is the surgeon who remarked casually, "Everybody knows that Orientals have a naturally higher threshold of pain than Occidentals. They don't feel pain as much as other races, that's why acupuncture works for them." Coming from a prestigious medical man, this statement would completely discourage most people from even considering acupuncture. In response to such remarks about acupuncture, you should know that in a 1977 pain-threshold experiment using Occidental and Oriental subjects, measurements of acupuncture-induced pain relief did *not* reflect race, but only individual human differences. Contrary to the stereotype cited by the surgeon, Oriental subjects showed more distress in one pain test than did the Occidentals. In fact, United States patients of various ethnic backgrounds—among others African, Hispanic and Native American—have received effective acupuncture treatment.

It is frequently suggested that you have to believe in acupuncture for it to work. You don't, any more than you have to believe in antibiotics or painkillers for them to work: that is, to have an observable, measurable effect on you. Belief that treatment of any kind will do some good, helps; but it's not the whole story. Most of us have experienced the *placebo effect,* estimated to produce from 30% to 40% of the value of any therapy. A placebo is a non-medication pill, or fake medication, which produces a physical benefit. Don't laugh—European doctors have had this useful trick up their sleeves at least since the 17th century. It is not magic. The toothache which goes away when you reach the dentist's office is an example of the placebo effect at work. How often have you said, "It hurt when I made the appointment," and wondered if the trip was necessary, until examination revealed tooth decay? If you are treated by 3 doctors in the same specialty and with equal qualifications, you generally do better with the one who inspires your confidence and trust. This also is the placebo effect at work.

Morphine relieves servere pain about 75% of the time. Because clinical experience and observation suggest 35% of that relief may be due to the placebo effect, medical scientists investigated brain chemistry to learn what accounts for it. They found that taking medication, or receiving treatment which you expect will ease your pain, triggers production of brain chemicals which effect the body, mind and emotions very much like a pharmaceutical—manufactured—drug. Therefore, a general standard applied to evaluating therapies is that 50% relief or more means that treatment itself is effective, aside from any placebo effect. Because relief as reported by patients can't be measured with absolute specificity, down to 1% or 3%, the 50% is a guideline, not a rigid law.

* * *

An internist in his late fifties who visited China on a doctors' tour in 1981 talked about observing acupuncture in hospitals and clinics.

"I've been very impressed by what I've seen. I cannot explain it from my own medical knowledge, but I think it should be investigated further. You know, we doctors are almost a closed-minded people, and we really don't want to hear about acupuncture, by and large."

Speaking of the firm grip of medical fashion, he added, "We all get locked into certain techniques. If something happens to a patient, and you haven't followed the particular technique that is accepted by the medical community, you may have a nice little malpractice suit."

For a perspective on medical dictates, consider a statement by the father of United States medicine, Dr. Benjamin Rush, who died in 1813. Dr. Rush reflected the prevailing views of his colleagues when he insisted that patients with any kind of disease should be purged and bled. In 1843 this practice was declared to be nonsense.

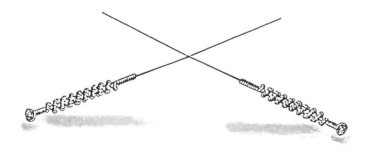

TWO

Acupuncture Therapy— Applications and Limitations

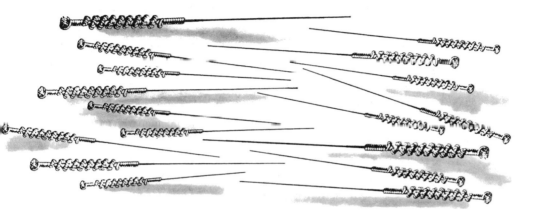

ACUPUNCTURE is not medication, like tetracycline or aspirin. It is a system of health care. Like other medical systems it aims to prevent and cure disease and thus prolong life. Acupuncture is applied in a more limited way in the United States than in China, where both Western medicine and Traditional medicine are official systems practiced in hospitals. Western medicine was firmly established in China long before the 1950s when Traditional medicine was incorporated into China's public health administration. Today, the medical student in China training for a career in acupuncture follows a curriculum which is one-third Western medicine—including biochemistry, physiology and pathology—and two-thirds Traditional medicine. The student working for a doctorate in Western medicine follows a reverse course of roughly one-third Traditional medicine. In practice, a surgeon trained in a Chinese school of Western medicine often works with an acupuncture-trained anesthetist.

In the United States professional cooperation between practitioners of different medical systems is highly unusual. For research purposes, some university medical schools have set up acupuncture clinics on a temporary basis. Otherwise, acupuncture is not generally available in hospital settings.

The status of acupuncture sets practical limits on the kinds of health problems suitable for acupuncture treatment in this country. For example, in China many cases have been recorded of successful treatment of acute appendicitis with acupuncture, without surgery. However, the patients were hospitalized. Their response to treatment was closely monitored. If acupuncture proved ineffective, they could be moved into surgery before the appendix ruptured. It would be utterly foolish in the United States to seek acupuncture treatment of acute appendicitis instead of standard medical treatment. The Chinese use acupuncture because it works. In cases which fail to respond adequately they are fully prepared to use Western medicine.

Another difference between what can be done with acupuncture in the United States and what is successfully treated in China, is the acceptability of techniques required for good results. An example is the Chinese treatment of paralysis following stroke. Scalp-needling, a technique developed in 1973, is particularly effective in cases of neurological damage. If therapy begins early, paralysis can be reversed; but treatment is reportedly painful.

Modification of treatment also makes a difference between the way acupuncture is applied in China, and its use in the United States. Acupuncture needles are twirled or otherwise manipulated to intensify stimulus. Strong stimulation can reduce the number of treatments needed; but may be uncomfortable, although not usually electrifyingly painful. Treatment in China tends to be more vigorous than that applied to Occidental patients in the United States, who have not been conditioned by lifelong awareness of this therapy. Think how conditioning affects your response to medical procedures. From infancy most of us have been used to hypodermic injections. We expect the pain, but we know from experience it doesn't last long.

People who are used to receiving acupuncture can accept treatment using strong stimulus. If the likelihood of success depends on strong stimulus, the patient's signs, symptoms and constitution must be evaluated to decide if acupuncture is suitable therapy. Just because you've read about some dramatic cure reported from China doesn't necessarily mean that your own similar case can be treated effectively in the United States.

Acupuncture is applied more broadly—for a wider range of ailments—in China, Japan and some European countries than it is in the United States. Doctors here rarely suggest acupuncture to their patients, and then only for a limited range of problems.

A well trained competent acupuncturist will tell you if your condition is suitable for acupuncture treatment; if Western medication is appropriate; or if a combination of therapies is indicated.

* * *

Many people ask, *is acupuncture safe?* As a health care system acupuncture has some inherent safeguards. Because treatment is drug free, you avoid taking one medication for ten days only to find it's not working, so you have to try a different dosage, or another drug. Some drugs take three weeks to test and then eliminate from the system before trying another.

Acupuncture treatment can be adjusted during a session because your response tells the acupuncturist if correct points have been chosen, or if a different combination of points should be used. Acupuncture allows continuous immediate examination of the patient's reaction: treatment is diagnostic as well as therapeutic.

Acupuncture does not mask underlying pathology. Headaches, for example, come in many shapes and sizes. Some start at the back of the neck, some at the temples, others across the top of the head. Some accompany fever, or nausea; others mean you're getting a cold. Headaches and associated symptoms hit you differently depending on what causes the headache. A migraine, or a sinus headache, can usually be relieved by acupuncture. But such headaches normally are part of a recurring condition. Unless proper and sufficient treatment is given to correct underlying causes of migraine and sinus problems, these headaches will return.

We often suffer from more than one ailment at a time. To avoid additional symptoms, prescribed medications must be compatible with each other. Because acupuncture is not medication, you can be treated for more than one condition in a session. For example, some hypertension responds to acupuncture. A patient with this condition who wants treatment to quit smoking can have simultaneous treatment for both problems: treating one does not interfere with treating the other.

With drugs, people often develop *tolerance*—the need for increased dosage to achieve the same required effect. This does not happen with acupuncture.

As with conventional medicine, the patient's ability to follow directions affects the safety of acupuncture treatment. Haven't you heard people say, "The doctor said to take two, but I figure I'll take four and really knock this thing out of my system?"

One acupuncturist told of a patient whom he had left in the treatment room after telling her to lie still until he returned. "The next thing I knew," he said, "she appeared fully dressed in the waiting room!"

Controlling his dismay, he calmly escorted her back to the treatment room, persuaded her to take off the necessary garments, girdle included, and was vastly relieved to note that all 12 needles were easily removable: luckily not one had bent or broken.

Sometimes small needles with flat circular handles are set into the ear and taped into place. You are told to press the needle from time to time, and to keep the needled ear dry. A similar treatment uses surgical steel staples, which you are instructed to jiggle with a clean finger. Staples don't require tape to secure them. Your finger comes into direct contact with pierced skin. Dirt on the finger could cause infection. In either case failure to follow directions can complicate treatment.

Some patients don't think of telling the acupuncturist that they are on medication. If you regularly take corticoids for respiratory problems; betablockers for a heart condition; or follow any long- or short-term drug regime, even a brief course of antibiotics for infection, tell your acupuncturist.

People starting acupuncture treatment have different reasons for not mentioning medication. A common reason is that the medication is for a different condition than the one which brings you to acupuncture. Or you may think of acupuncture as so remote from the system which produced your prescription that there is no interaction. But some hormones, especially opposite-sex hormones, reduce the effect of acupuncture. You should also know that acupuncture intensifies the effect of some drugs. This is why dosage can be reduced during a course of acupuncture treatment, and why some medications may even be eliminated. However, any reduction must take place gradually, in consultation with the acupuncturist and the prescribing doctor.

It has happened that a patient decided to stop taking medication for a week or so before starting acupuncture treatment. The motive may have been, "I'm starting a whole new approach, so I'll start with a clean slate." This may be good philosophy when you change jobs or move to a new house; but it is not applicable to your health care. Abrupt withdrawal of a drug to which your system has adapted can be devastating, if not fatal. Never go cold turkey off a prescription drug regimen!

You can help yourself get the greatest benefit from acupuncture by calling attention to any unusual aspects of the way you live. Your special activities might make 'permanent' needles inadvisable. For example, someone who swims daily would probably not be treated with press needles to be worn for a week.

✳ ✳ ✳

Can acupuncture harm you? Should some people avoid this system of health care?

Properly administered, acupuncture does no harm. However, certain conditions should be brought to the acupuncturist's attention so that treatment may be modified to suit the patient. If you have a cardiac pacemaker, and want acupuncture treatment for sinus problems, a back injury or sciatica—some of the problems for which electrically enhanced acupuncture is often used—the acupuncturist will avoid this form of stimulation because of possible electro-magnetic interference with the pacemaker.

Tell the acupuncturist if there's any chance that you are pregnant. Points normally used for certain conditions stimulate contractions of the uterus. Other points can be substituted for these contraction-stimulating ones. However, because of risk of inducing abortion, many acupuncturists prefer not to treat a woman in early stages of pregnancy. Some will not treat a pregnant woman at all.

If you have a tendency to hemorrhage, or are a diagnosed hemophiliac, acupuncture is not for you.

Some previous modes of treatment can interfere temporarily with your ability to respond to acupuncture. Certain medications affect response to acupuncture. Also, surgical scars may short-circuit the response mechanism. However, experienced practitioners know how to work around the obstacle presented by a scar.

Some people show little or no reaction to acupuncture. One physician-acupuncturist claims there are no people with natural resistance to this therapy. In his opinion, treatment fails only because it has not been correctly applied. Another equally experienced physician-acupuncturist states that 5%-15% of patients don't respond to acupuncture. An eminent acupuncturist-teacher insists that acupuncture will always help a patient if the practitioner is good. Some acupuncturists tell you that if there is no response after 6 treatments you are unlikely to benefit from acupuncture. Others say the same thing using different figures— 8, 12 or 14. So far no absolute standards have been established to describe who responds and who does not.

A woman in her early fifties had suffered since her teens from chronic back pain. She described the condition as "an unstable back with spurs." She tried acupuncture at the suggestion of a neurologist in whom she had great faith. After the first treatment she felt sudden relief, and enthusiastically walked ten blocks home. By the time she arrived, her back hurt again. During the next 3 weeks she had 6 treatments which produced no significant improvement, so she quit.

When he was about fifty, this patient's brother tried acupuncture for an acute problem—frozen shoulder. He did not know about his sister's acupuncture experience. He felt some relief after 3 treatments, but it didn't last. There was still no real improvement after 6 treatments. His physician-acupuncturist said that acupuncture doesn't help everyone, and terminated treatment. Neither patient had any adverse effects.

No method of health care can guarantee 100% success If well-performed acupuncture has no effect on you, you'll be disappointed but not damaged: in itself, lack of reaction is not harmful.

Are there health problems for which acupuncture is definitely not recommended? Any health emergency demands immediate standard medical attention, because time is vitally important. Problems which can signal medical emergency are: pain or pressure in chest or upper abdomen; difficulty in breathing, or shortness of breath; fainting or feeling faint; dizziness, sudden weakness or a severe pain anywhere in the body.

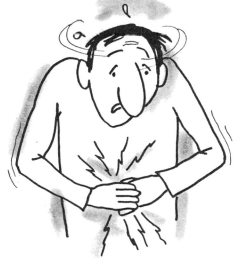

As an example, acute abdominal pain often signals a problem needing surgery, like peritonitis or acute appendicitis.

Conventional treatment of acute appendicitis is routinely so successful that there is no benefit in seeking alternative methods. The famous James Reston case, which drew United States public attention to acupuncture in 1971, involved acupuncture treatment to relieve severe postoperative pain *following* appendectomy. This use of acupuncture is not generally available to U.S. hospital patients.

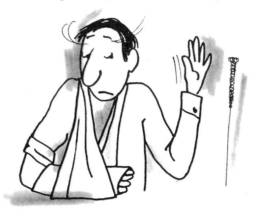

If you break a bone, it should be treated conventionally. However, because acupuncture improves circulation it could be useful in the healing period, provided the necessary points are accessible and not hidden under a cast.

Structural damage resulting from organic problems will not yield to acupuncture. For example, a fully formed cataract—resulting from chemical changes in the protein of the eye lens—cannot be helped by acupuncture. The cataract must be surgically removed. Inguinal hernia, in which part of the intestine protrudes through a gap in abdominal wall muscles, usually near the groin, must be surgically repaired by joining muscle fibers so that the bulging section of intestine is made to stay in its normal place. Acupuncture cannot accomplish this structural repair.

Most experts agree that other conditions unsuitable for acupuncture treatment are: severe infectious diseases; any form of cancer; congestive heart failure; and paralysis which has lasted more than two years.

✳ ✳ ✳

When people ask *what diseases can be treated by acupuncture,* it's like saying, "Tell me what acupuncture can do for everything from Acne to Herpes Zoster." How would the question sound in the framework of Western medicine? With conventional medicine very few health care questions can be sufficiently answered by a simple "yes" or "no." You know how often answers include the phrase, "it depends." Any experienced and honest doctor is sure to have told you that predicted response to a course of treatment is subject to variables. You will hear the same from an experienced and honest acupuncturist.

Acupuncture can be effective treatment for some patients with a particular cluster of *signs*—clues to disease that can be observed, and *symptoms*—feelings reported by the patient; yet less effective for other patients with similar signs and symptoms. (Vomiting is a sign; nausea, a symptom.)

In considering acupuncture you want to know if your specific health condition can be helped by this form of treatment. Why would acupuncture be good for you as a patient? These questions can't be answered by ticking off items on a shopping list of diseases according to whether or not a certain ailment is known to have responded to acupuncture.

From the acupuncture point of view no two patients present identical combinations of signs, symptoms, history and constitution. You may be a vigorous businesswoman in your mid-fifties, beginning to limp because from time to time your left hip hurts badly; or a fairly sedentary scholar whose big toe sometimes causes such pain that you can hardly walk from your desk to the bookshelf; or a rural mail carrier seriously hampered by low-back pain; or a frail elderly single person whose aching fingers can barely turn the doorkey. The general label *rheumatism* may be put on the condition of each of these four people. But just as no two adults have identical fingerprints, so do their 'health fingerprints' vary. Each of these four people works and lives differently, and has a different emotional outlook and level of vitality from the others. The acupuncture patient is treated according to the unique pattern presented by her or his collection of signs, symptoms, health history and constitution—the patient's special blend of strengths and weaknesses.

Even though acupuncture is not yet a routine form of treatment in the United States, a broad range of ailments has been treated effectively. Benefits range from modest satisfactory improvement to great improvement with long-term relief. As a general rule acupuncture works best on *musculoskeletal* problems; in cases of *impaired physiology*—ailments in which bodily processes don't work properly; and conditions in which *pain* is the chief symptom.

This grouping of health problems is useful for an orderly discussion of disease, but you know that disease is a disorderly condition. There is often a domino effect in sickness, with one complaint—and, sometimes, the attempts to cure it—prompting the appearance of another.

Under each heading a few diseases are listed to give you an idea of the kinds of problems which have been helped by acupuncture. These lists are neither exhaustive nor exclusive. They are samples. If you decide to try acupuncture, the acupuncturist will tell you if your problem is suitable for treatment.

Musculoskeletal Problems

This category includes osteoarthritis and rheumatoid arthritis; joint pains of unknown origin; low-back problems; sprains in arms, hands, legs and feet; stiff neck; and tendosynovitis—inflammation of the tendon-sheath lining.

Acupuncture cannot reverse destructive bone changes caused by advanced osteoarthritis, nor relocate a slipped disk. It can stimulate circulation, relieve muscle spasm, and reduce swelling. Signs of the disease may still show in X-ray pictures; but reduction of symptoms makes all the difference in the quality of your daily life.

Impaired Physiology

Allergies include asthma, eczema, hayfever, hives and sinus problems. A person subject to allergic reactions can present different

signs at different times. One woman in her thirties suffers season-
ally from hayfever, with runny nose, sneezing, and watering eyes.
During the last year, not in her usual hayfever season, she noted
that after wearing a gold necklace for several hours her skin showed
clear marks as if the necklace had been etched on it. The necklace
is 14 kt. gold and she had worn it often without such a reaction.
Acupuncture theory makes a close connection between upper-
respiratory tract allergic signs and skin problems. Acupuncture
can modify the reaction to antigens—substances whose stimulus
to the system causes a variety of allergic signs.

Circulation involves blood vessels, and is, of course,
associated with the heart. In acupuncture the heart itself is never
directly treated with needles. However, acupuncture can be effective for some nervous conditions which affect the heart. These
include angina pectoris; bradycardia—slow heartbeat; palpitations—fast powerful beating of the heart; and tachycardia—
extremely rapid heartbeat. Ischemia—deficient blood supply,
signs of which are cold hands and feet—responds to acupuncture's
ability to increase circulation. Acupuncture cannot erase varicose
veins, but can eliminate the accompanying aches, stinging and
cramps.

Gastrointestinal problems afflict people whose digestive systems tremble constantly on the verge of disorder. Constipation; chronic gastritis—stomach inflammation; diarrhea; dyspep-
sia—indigestion; gallbladder inflammation; hemorrhoids; and
peptic ulcer disease are some gastrointestinal afflictions which
acupuncture can alleviate. As with varicose veins, which they
resemble, hemorrhoids cannot be structurally repaired by
acupuncture; but this treatment can ease pain and discomfort.

Some ailments develop when impaired physiology
causes the body to over-produce a natural substance. In peptic
ulcer disease the stomach is stimulated to produce too much acid.
This bitter substance overwhelms protective mucus and eats away
at your digestive tract. If the process goes on long enough a hole,
or ulcer, appears. Medication can heal a developed ulcer, a job
which acupuncture can't do. However, if begun early enough in

the course of this disease, acupuncture can rebalance body processes and ward off development of the ulcer by establishing and maintaining the right proportion of mucus to acid.

Genitourinary problems which can be helped by acupuncture include impotence; kidney disorders; menstrual dysfunction; prostatitis; and urinary tract infections.

Acupuncture-assisted childbirth is unusual in this country, but patients who have managed to arrange for it would repeat the experience. Acupuncture strengthens uterine contractions, reduces maternal blood loss, and lowers the degree of stress on the fetus, while reducing the mother's pain.

Chronic headaches are a special category of illness. Acupuncture has given effective relief and long-term remission of migraines, sinus headaches and tension headaches. Patients usually come to acupuncture for relief of persistent, recurring headache after extensive conventional diagnosis has failed to show any underlying pathology. In many cases a course of acupuncture treatment has reduced the frequency of headaches; or has given long-term relief.

Nerve problems include facial palsy; intercostal neuralgia—severe pain between the ribs; sciatica; and shingles—a very painful rash which occurs when a dormant chicken-pox virus (herpes zoster) is jostled awake years after you had this classic childhood disease. Continued pain after the viral infection disappears is called post-herpetic neuralgia. It can attack the face as well as the body. In addition to these nerve problems, some results of stroke, like facial and other paralysis, have also responded well to acupuncture.

Addiction involves brain activities which are remarkably similar no matter what the substance of addiction is. Problems of addiction to food and tobacco have responded well to acupuncture treatment, which reinforces your motivation to lose weight and/or stop smoking. Acupuncture can reduce signs and symptoms of alcohol- and narcotics-withdrawal; but most alcoholics and drug addicts need supportive services along with treatment, in order to conquer their habits.

Cosmetic acupuncture can restore tone, and give a more youthful appearance, to aging facial skin by increasing circulation and stimulating underlying muscles.

Pain

Most diseases bring pain and misery, so you may wonder why pain is a separate category of conditions suitable for acupuncture treatment.

Not every disease involves a great deal of long-lasting pain. Cystitis—inflammation of the urinary bladder more common in women than in men gives you the feeling that you constantly need to urinate. The feeling persists even after you've emptied your bladder.

"It's a colossal nuisance, and a constant source of tension and discomfort and anxiety," says a woman who has suffered recurring bouts of cystitis, "but it's not really painful."

In many disorders, however, pain is the chief complaint.

There is useful pain and useless pain. Useful pain helps us survive: it makes you pull away from flames or hot surfaces; it tells you that your bare foot has stepped on a thumbtack. If we didn't feel pain we'd walk around with sharp objects piercing our skin, inviting infection; incur many blisters, which also attract infection; never know when we've damaged a bone or joint; and be unaware of organic problems requiring medical attention.

Not all pain signals that damage has occurred. Some pain outlives its purpose.

As anyone who has endured it knows, **severe chronic pain** makes it hard to focus on anything beyond the pain which surrounds and fills you. You distort your posture to avoid moving in certain ways that can trigger a pain crisis. You sleep badly because shifting position may awaken the pain. Poor sleep and anxiety about the next attack of pain cause depression. Another source of depression is the worry about taking painkilling medication—will you need it the rest of your life? Pain sets up a vicious cycle: it hurts to move, so you move less; limiting your motion reduces circulation and encourages neural actions which cause more pain; and less activity means more disability. Damned if you move and damned if you don't—no wonder some chronic pain sufferers become suicidal.

Some chronic pain is the legacy of an old injury; some is a disease symptom. However, most chronic pain, persistent or sporadic, is not a signal, it is the main health problem of the person suffering it.

In the early 1970s pain became the topic of much basic and applied research. Also in this period, scientific investigators were looking for concrete explanations of acupuncture analgesia: how was acupuncture able to block pain well enough for major surgery to be performed on conscious patients? These separate lines of inquiry were sometimes linked by shared professional interests.

The 1970s also saw the establishment of centers for comprehensive treatment of pain, where physicians work with other types of health care professionals for the benefit of a pretty desperate class of patient. Many people are referred to such centers by doctors who have organized multiple assaults on a patient's pain without establishing a beach-head, because nothing works.

At these centers many approaches to pain treatment are tried: bio-feedback, nutrition, transcutaneous electro-nerve-stimulation (TENS) and hypnotherapy, among others. Because of its recognized effectiveness in reducing chronic pain, acupuncture is usually an option for patients at comprehensive pain management centers.

One course of acupuncture treatment rarely gives longlasting or permanent relief of chronic pain: repeated courses may be needed. However, the pain-relieving effect of acupuncture accumulates; so even if you need more treatment, later courses generally require fewer sessions than the first series. Some chronic pain patients eventually become pain free. Others may need several treatments a year; but can live comfortably with reduced medication, or none. If you have endured great pain for a long time, 60%-70% reduction of pain makes a real difference. The improvement in how you feel reduces the anxiety which is such a large part of pain; and frees many people from the depression which clouded their existence in a state of pain.

Attacks of **acute severe pain** also respond well to acupuncture. The normal recovery period from back spasm is about eight weeks. Pain and stiffness of frozen shoulder can last for months. Tennis elbow—a painful inflammation afflicting violinists and cellists as well as amateur athletes—can last six months. The fact that these conditions are self-limiting is little comfort to the sufferer. These problems are recent events without long-tern history; and acupuncture often relieves them relatively quickly.

Trigeminal neuralgia, a facial pain sometimes called *tic douloureux*, responds very well to acupuncture if treated early, and if it has not previously been treated by surgery.

The use of acupuncture in dentistry is common in China, but very limited in the United States. Some patients report preferring acupuncture to novocaine.

Remember, the diseases listed are samples only. They typify the category under which they are listed. If your particular health problem is not listed, it is easy enough to decide if it fits into the musculoskeletal group, the impaired physiology group, or the pain group. Only you can decide if you are comfortable enough with the treatment you are receiving; or if you want to explore the possible benefits of a different mode of treatment.

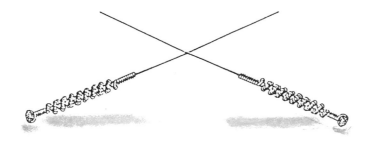

THREE

The Acupuncturist and Case Notes

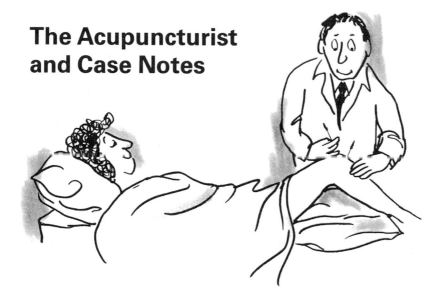

YOU have decided to try acupuncture. How do you find the right practitioner for you?

Acupuncturists work in various settings: individual or group private practice; medical center pain clinic; independent comprehensive pain clinics; and alternative health centers. Convenience affects your choice of setting, which may be limited outside urban areas.

Acupuncturists recognize the need for patient-education. You can generally get some basic information by telephoning; and many practitioners give an initial free consultation. In any case, consultation is usual before you embark upon treatment.

Just as you would with a new doctor, start picking up clues to how the acupuncturist you are about to consult manages patients.

A woman with such acute sciatic pain that she needed a metal brace to walk, was referred by a friend to an acupuncturist. She described her condition to him over the telephone. Arriving at his suburban office for the first appointment, she faced a steep hillside climb up a flight of stairs equivalent to four floors of a city building.

"I suppose this builds character," she thought as she struggled to the top. "Besides, these acupuncturists probably do things differently from other people."

By contrast, the acupuncturist who posts a sign in the waiting room to explain the odor of burning *moxa*—an herb used in some treatment—reveals sensitivity to the inexperienced patient. For every person entranced by fumes of smoldering herb, there's another who takes offense.

You arrive on time for your appointment; the waiting room is full.

"We're running late," the receptionist says brightly.

Is this a sign that the practitioner is eminent, heavily in demand, and therefore superior in every way? Is it a subtle insult from a health care professional who undervalues the patient's time? Does it show the kind of management which makes patients complain of assembly-line handling in which you rarely see the same acupuncturist twice? Answers to the first two questions depend on your point of view.

An answer to the third question has practical consequences. In a course of treatment it is better for you to be seen by no more than two acupuncturists, rather than by a different one each time, as can happen in a large group practice. Ideas of which points to treat for your complaint can vary, as can styles of manipulating needles. If several acupuncturists work on one patient during a treatment series, inconsistency may result; this can confuse the body's responses. Unified treatment serves the patient best.

The relatively informal environment of some alternative health care offices relaxes one patient; while another, nervously venturing outside conventional medicine, is reassured to find practitioner and staff wearing white, just like the doctors who failed to cure this patient of *tic douloureux*. We are not machines: our responses to environment vary a great deal.

Is there informational literature on display? Does the

atmosphere put you at ease? The waiting room doesn't tell the whole story, but it offers useful clues.

If you're like most people who come to acupuncture after other remedies have failed, you're looking for relief, not diagnosis. The general pattern is that new acupuncture patients have been seen by several doctors whose diagnoses agree. Such patients usually have tried many forms of treatment which either failed to give long-term relief, or produced undesirable side effects.

A woman in her early thirties was diagnosed as having systemic lupus erythematosus, an autoimmune condition with signs that include skin eruptions, fever, blood poisoning and kidney damage.

"Doctors were very pessimistic when I got it," she said, adding that she had been thoroughly diagnosed. "I went to so many doctors, I kept looking for one who didn't want me to take preventive cortisone." This was ten years ago. Discussing her results with acupuncture treatment, she said, "I've been immensely cured by it; I feel very optimistic even though I still have lupus: if I go out in the sun or mistreat my body, I get sick. But I haven't gone into crisis, I'm leading a perfectly normal life, due to acupuncture."

Amply diagnosed in conventional medical terms, you're still walking or limping or shuffling around with your problem. If you're trying acupuncture because your doctor referred you—most likely in cases of intractable pain without organic cause—you've probably brought along a copy of the diagnosis. However, unless required by state regulation, or by your health insurance, it is unnecessary to bring a medical commentary on your condition: diagnosis is very much part of the acupuncturist's training. Diagnosis may be carried out by traditional Chinese methods, Western-medicine methods, or a combination of the two. Medical systems differ, but the stage for medical performance is the same—the human body, mind and emotions. Western pulse-taking and Chinese pulse-taking differ; but close observation of the patient is crucial to both systems of health care.

In the initial consultation you will learn if your complaint is known to respond to acupuncture; and approximately how many treatments you will need. The nature of your problem, the length of time you've had it, your age and general health all affect response to treatment.

Fees average $30. per visit, with regional variations. One woman who had shyly refrained from asking, wondered in mid-treatment if she was to be charged by the needle. No—you are charged by the treatment.

During consultation, try to form an idea of the practitioner's overall treatment style. Variations are played on the theme of acupuncture in the United States. Some acupuncturist will be more in tune with your needs than others.

Early Chinese medical writings described diagnosis of the patient's mental and emotional, as well as physical, condition. From an acupuncture perspective, you don't have physical problems without affecting your mind and emotions; and you don't have mental or emotional disorders without some physical effect. A vogue word has been borrowed from philosophy to label this way of diagnosing and treating patients: 'holistic.' Thirty years ago in a small coastal Maine town, the local doctor practiced holistic medicine: he had to—there were no specialists available to his hardworking patients. To go back further, Sir William Osler, who founded the Johns Hopkins Medical School, and has been called 'the father of Western scientific medicine', took what is now called the holistic view when he said, "It is not so much the kind of disease the patient has, as the kind of patient who has the disease, which must be asked."

Osler, a Canadian, learned acupuncture from a British colleague. Osler wrote of using it successfully to treat lumbago and sciatica. However, he never described acupuncture as a Chinese form of treatment. Scholars believe he was unfamiliar with its origin.

Recently an eminent Chinese acupuncturist, sounding very much like Osler, said, "The patient is the focus of our health care."

One acupuncturist may proceed briskly but thoroughly

from interview to treatment. After years of observing patients, an experienced acupuncturist can keep questions to a minimum. Another practitioner may ask more questions than you think suitable coming from anyone but a psychotherapist. Some acupuncture training emphasises extensive questioning of the patient.

Twenty-nine acupuncture schools were founded in the United States, beginning in the early 1970s. Some require, or urge, students to take part of their studies, or continuing professional education courses, abroad. But the work is based on the same body of knowledge, even when tradition or style varies from one school to another. By analogy, both Bach and the Beatles composed and played Western music, but used it differently. Variations on the theme of acupuncture are a matter of emphasis.

Experienced practitioners treat at the level of the patient's expressed need.

"We were taught not to treat symptoms," said an acupuncturist with a private practice in Florida, "but after a few years in practice, you recognize that for some patients, symptomatic treatment is what they're asking for, and it's suitable at that time."

Classical acupuncture texts say that body, mind and emotion are inseparable: what injures one, affects the other two. This idea is not exotic: Western medicine held the same view until the 17th century, when Cartesian philosophy promoted belief in the separation of human mind and matter; and laid the groundwork for our common experience of medical practice as a jigsaw puzzle of specialists. Western physicians are perfectly aware that body, mind and emotions are interdependent. However, the realities of our modern Western medical system make it unlikely that one doctor will treat you extensively for both depression and low-back pain.

When you've lived with a painful lower back, and it finally stops hurting, your disposition is bound to improve. However some patients have reported that effects of acupuncture transcended pain relief by healing them in unexpected ways. These people said that, during treatment of a musculo-skeletal problem, needling at one point produced such a sensation of emotional relief that they wept. Such episodes marked the beginning of improved emotional well-being. These profound healing experiences occurred whether or not the practitioner was trained according to theories emphasizing a deep psychotherapeutic approach to illness.

✳ ✳ ✳

M. sued her employer, a large corporation, on a sex-discrimination issue. She won her case, but after the trial she slipped into emotional and physical decline. Suffering from severe panic attacks and nightmares, she shook and sweated constantly. She was unable to work, and began to feel suicidal. M. tried various therapies: fear clinic, dietary changes, hypnosis, meditation, yoga and drugs. Except for meditation, which she stopped after 3 months, everything helped a little; but the phobic symptoms continued to interfere with her life.

M. went to an acupuncturist for treatment of a condition unrelated to her phobic problems. She did, however, mention them to the practitioner. He said he could cure the panic attacks. She was skeptical, but willing to try this unfamiliar application of acupuncture.

M. reported that 6 months later she felt like a different person. The panic attacks stopped completely; she was able to return to work; the treatment helped her "come to terms with the [lawsuit] experience and other traumas and has helped me transform my inner life completely. Acupuncture gave me my life back."

✳ ✳ ✳

A. felt confused and under stress after several months of rough experiences. She did not want to take medication; or to enter a course of psychotherapy. She needed help, but wasn't sure what kind. She heard of a reputable acupuncture clinic, and decided to have a treatment.

"Within five minutes a strange sensation came over me. Deep inside my chest area I felt a shaking and shuddering that was uncontrollable. It was as if some little person was running around and around inside my body and making everything shake and bang about. I also felt as if somebody had opened a tap and piles of tension and stress was pouring out and just making my body shake in its hurry to get out."

After 20 minutes the acupuncturist returned, and asked how she felt. A. related her experience and said she felt good; the acupuncturist adjusted needles and left again. "A similar pattern of events took place with the shakes but much milder."

Later that day, she recalled, "the calm and grief I felt was very noticeable. It was not as if I had jogged 5 miles or had just had a good massage, but a calmness *inside*. There was no more tension coming from deep inside. I felt as if 6 months of stress that had built up had gone. Stress and tension was not a concern for several months after treatment."

✳ ✳ ✳

A psychiatrist who now practices acupuncture fulltime said, "I do very little psychotherapy, the needles themselves do it. You must trust them." In his practice, he has had "a lot of success with eating disorders, and with depression. A small amount of touching the psyche makes ripples which can last for months."

People who enter conventional Western psychotherapy for emotional problems often find that physical ailments are alleviated in the course of treatment. In a different sequence of healing, patients who seek relief of physical ailments often find emotional, as well as physical, relief through acupuncture. Scientific studies suggest that the sense of well-being produced by acupuncture is associated with release of brain chemicals. While this may not be a complete explanation, the effect is easily observable in veterinary acupuncture. (Animals can't discuss their feelings—behavior reveals them.) A large dog, yawning and dozing while acupuncture needles project from his back and paws, is the picture of relaxation. The human patient often experiences similar relief of tension.

Your temperament and your health problems determine

what you want from treatment. Sometimes you simply want effective drug free treatment of bothersome signs and symptoms. In different circumstances you might need treatment of underlying causes, a deeper kind of healing. Sometimes you feel the need for a profound change in your life: you might prefer a practitioner who emphasizes psychotherapeutic possibilities of acupuncture.

The practitioner's overall treatment style reflects training, philosophy, experience and personality. Consultation is not commitment on your part. You may want to see other acupuncturists and compare procedures, overall treatment styles, and fees. You may also want to go away and think some more about acupuncture. No responsible acupuncturist will pressure you to enter treatment.

* * *

Acupuncture regulation varies from state to state. You may have to sign a declaration of informed consent before receiving treatment. This requirement dismays some people who reason that routine treatment by an M.D. or dentist can be given without having the patient sign such a form; therefore acupuncture must be riskier than conventional treatment. In fact, some people conclude that acupuncture must be as hazardous as an operation under general anesthesia, for which such written consent is always required. The demand for consent forms, in states which regulate acupuncture, reflects the conventional medical view of acupuncture as *experimental,* which it is not. What *is* experimental is Western scientific investigation aimed at explaining how acupuncture works. You are not signing up to be a guinea pig!

"The last time anybody put a needle into me was for a tetanus shot—I'm not kidding, it *hurt*!" the strong young man exclaimed, shuddering at the idea of acupuncture.

Acupuncture is *not at all* like being inoculated. Acupuncture needles are fine as thread, 1/3 to 1/4 the thickness of a hypodermic needle. They are solid, not hollow. In acupuncture the needles themselves are the treatment; they are not a way of pumping medicine into you. (Much of the ache and discomfort you feel after getting a shot is caused by the injected substance, as well as by the thickness of the hypodermic needle.) The standard acupuncture needle is stainless steel, with a shaft about 2 inches long. The straight handle is wire-wrapped or incised, so it can be gripped firmly for twirling or other manipulations which enhance the acupuncture effect. Special purpose needles, including flat circular press needles, come in various sizes.

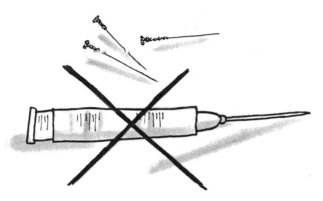

Either during consultation or at the first treatment, your blood pressure is taken. First-time patients often show a rise in blood pressure. If you are nervous about the acupuncture procedure, don't hesitate to say so. It's a perfectly natural response to trying unfamiliar treatment.

If you have come for treatment of a musculoskeletal problem, and also have hypertension, needling at the appropriate points for hypertension will be part of your treatment.

For acupuncture, you don't automatically take off your clothes and put on a robe. The amount of undressing required depends on the area the acupuncturist plans to treat.

A relaxed position is best for receiving acupuncture: you will most likely be asked to lie on a treatment table; although sometimes a patient is treated sitting.

It is standard practice to sterilize needles by high pressure steam, in an autoclave or pressure cooker. They are then wrapped in alcohol-soaked gauze. Many acupuncturists use disposable needles which come pre-sterlized in sealed packages.

The acupuncturist swabs your skin with alcohol before inserting sterilized needles. Some are placed in your painful area; others, at distant points. The acupuncturist will tell you not to move. A needle is pushed in far enough to locate the acupoint. Without looking, you can't tell if insertion is deep or shallow.

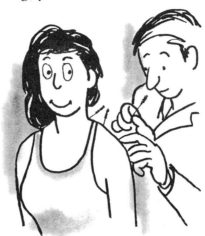

After a few needles had been placed in her hands, one inquisitive patient, lying on her back, raised her head to observe the procedure. She felt a quick mild stinging in her shoulder, and decided to follow orders.

If you move suddenly, you could bend a needle. Acupuncturists are trained to remove jammed, bent or broken needles; but it's better to avoid such problems, which disrupt treatment.

Besides first time anxiety, what do you feel? An experienced acupuncturist has a deft touch. You may not even feel some needles go in; with others you may feel a light prick, about like the jab of a sewing needle or splinter. Sensations peculiar to acupuncture come when the needle finds the acupoint: heaviness in the area around the needle; numbness; tingling; mild soreness; and something like a faint electric tickle running along your arm, leg or body from the point. The sensation—called *deqi*—is subjective and variable: you can benefit from treatment even if you haven't felt it. *Deqi* can be uncomfortable, but dies down in a few minutes.

Patients say it is a small price to pay for relief of the problem which brought them to acupuncture.

The acupuncturist may twirl the needle briefly, or move it up and down a little. These manipulations of the needle intensify the acupuncture sensation; they are done to strenghten treatment.

Strengthening treatment means making the action of the needles more powerful. The electric stimulator is a modern development replacing hand twirling of needles when this technique is needed for more than a minute or two. An electrode is attached to one or more needles. Wire runs from the electrode to a small machine with knobs and dials. The knobs control the pattern, frequency and strength of electrical impulses. What you feel is something like a tadpole twitching under your skin. If the twitch is too strong, ask to have it reduced. Treatment by electro-potentiated acupuncture needles can give noticeable relief of muscle spasm and sciatic pain, even in one session.

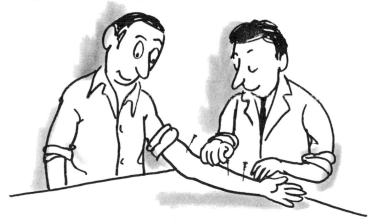

A traditional way of increasing the power of needles is moxibustion, in which a smoldering stick of moxa—the tropical herb *artemisia vulgaris*—warms the needles. In classical Chinese practice moxa, formed into small cones or pellets the size of a rice grain, is placed directly on an acupoint and allowed to burn down until it raises a blister. Sometimes a cone of moxa is set on a slice of ginger to burn down, thus producing indirect stimulation of the acupoint.

Treatment strength is commonly modified for American patients. This means that the acupuncturist will use several needles to produce an effect equal to one needle with powerful stimulation. Experience has shown that people for whom acupuncture is unusual therapy do better with more needles, and lighter stimulation spread over several treatments, than with very strong stimulation in one or two treatments. Frozen shoulder, for example, is a condition of unknown origin in which sudden severe pain is followed by stiffness which lasts several months. A very experienced acupuncturist can insert a six-inch needle and unfreeze the shoulder in a few minutes. You would feel strong discomfort, but not electrifying pain. The technique takes years to perfect, which is one reason it is seldom used. But the more powerful reason not to use it is to avoid frightening the patient. Different treatment, with more needles, may take longer; but for the majority of people who respond to acupuncture, needle therapy beats waiting months for the condition to clear up by itself.

In a treatment series, from time to time you'll probably note the acupuncturist using different combinations of points, or different needling techniques, or both. This means that new sources of healing are being stimulated in reply to the patient's response to treatment.

When the needles have been placed, the acupuncturist tells you to relax, then leaves to treat someone else.

"For the first time in years I wanted my mother," the college student said, laughing at the memory of how unnerved she was when left alone in the treatment room the first time she had acupuncture.

Another typical reaction is, 'What'll I do if I don't like this?'

Stop this little panic by recognizing that you are not alone in the desert. Remind yourself that all you have to do is call, and someone will come. List all the reasons you decided to try acupuncture. Sum up the disagreeable side effects of your most recent conventional treatment.

What usually happens is, you begin to relax and find

yourself wondering why you didn't ask how long this would take . . . funny, you can't feel the needles at all anymore . . . You may doze off, or float in the semi-awake state familiar to people who practice light meditation.

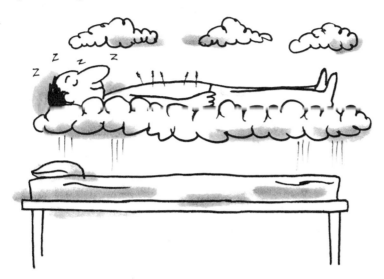

"After putting the needles in," one patient said, recalling his first acupuncture treatment, "the doctor wound a kitchen timer. I was surprised . . . and found it amusing."

If your acupuncturist uses this familiar device to time your treatment—a common, practical method—you may find the ticking is a reassuring domestic accompaniment to the waiting period. You may be startled when the timer goes off—how could you have fallen asleep?

The acupuncturist, or an assistant, comes back and removes the needles, swabbing your skin with alcohol. Except for some mild stinging caused by the alcohol, this procedure is painless. Try counting needles as they are removed. How many did you feel going in?

For some problems the effect of treatment is extended, after the needles have been removed, by having you lie with a heating pad on the trouble spot. Sometimes a medicated bandage is applied as additional treatment.

You may feel sleepy after acupuncture. This is not just the result of lying in a dimly-lit room for twenty minutes: acupuncture has a calming effect on many patients. People also often feel a sudden sense of well-being quite separate from the degree of pain relief. Enjoy this mild euphoria—it's harmless.

* * *

"In 1972, at my annual physical, I complained for the second year of a deep-seated pain under the lower inner corner of my right shoulder blade," said R., a journalist in his late fifties. "X-rays showed nothing. My doctor suggested acupuncture. At that time it was a pretty adventurous suggestion. Because of my respect for the doctor I agreed to try it, but I had no particular expectations. It would either work or not."

R. lives in New York City. His doctor referred him to a Chinese-American, the daughter and granddaughter of acupuncturists who had practiced in Shanghai.

"The acupuncturist herself set the number of treatments at our first meeting—eight. I went once a week. She used suction cups around the pain, as well as needles, some of which she twirled.

"I wrote the doctor after the last treatment that I was 75% improved.

"For a couple of years I had always looked for a straight chair when I went to someone's house. I always sat a certain way to accommodate the pain. Two months after the last treatment, I was sitting in my usual careful way when I suddenly thought, 'I wonder if I can sit in the easy chair over there.' I did. I realized the pain was gone. I'd had it for two years; but it hasn't come back in ten years."

R.'s story illustrates some useful things to remember about acupuncture.

- Acupuncture is effective even when your attitude toward it is neutral.
- Acupuncture subtly encourages the body's natural tendency to heal itself. Until stimulated by acupuncture, R.'s self-healing ca-

pacity had not been sufficient to overcome his back pain.

• Physiological processes stimulated by acupuncture continue to work after the immediate stimulus—the needle—is removed.

✻

G. is an urban planner, in private practice as a consultant. She was 41 when interviewed. She had a sinus condition, with sporadic severe headaches.

"Conventional treatment made me feel as if my body were invaded by drugs. Medication made me drowsy, and interfered with my work.

"My sister-in-law had been satisfied by acupuncture treatment, and suggested I try it for my sinus problem.

"I made an appointment with the acupuncturist who had treated my sister-in-law. By coincidence, I came down with a acute sinus headache the day I was to go to Chinatown for my first treatment. I went anyway, even though I sure didn't feel like making the trip all the way downtown.

"The acupuncturist was Chinese. His English wasn't wonderful, but his assistant helped with any language problem. He diagnosed by taking my pulse, looking at my eyes and throat, and asking questions.

"My attitude was, I was just going to give it a try. Even so, I was disappointed, when I left after treatment, to find that this headache was not miraculously gone."

Despite her disappointment, G. returned for more treatments. She had needles in her face, some of which were electro-stimulated. After each session of needle therapy, G. was given herbs, which she either "just took," or drank in water.

"They didn't have much taste . . . rather bland."

After three treatments G. felt better. The sinus condition cleared up completely after the fifth, and had not recurred when she was interviewed, four years after the last treatment.

G. also had a history of back trouble. She went to a

chiropractor, but her back continued to bother her. At 31 she had surgery to fuse two vertebrae.

"My back started acting up again in the winter of '81-'82. I called a back doctor who said, 'Well, we can always go in there again and fuse the next two.' I didn't like that idea. Back surgery was traumatic. The operation took a year out of my life.

"I saw a physiatrist—a doctor who specializes in physical medicine. I told him I was thinking of using acupuncture, which had worked well for my sinus. He was receptive to the idea, and said acupuncture had proven useful in arthritis."

G. returned to the acupuncturist.

"I felt some trepidation when I saw that he planned to use, among others, a 6″ needle. The ones he'd used for my sinus were less than half that long.

"I felt no particular pain when the needles were inserted. Some, I didn't even feel. There was a dullness and pressure that seemed to spread around the spot where the needle went in.

"During the period I was having back treatment, I thought I'd developed some kind of genito-urinary problem. The day I planned to mention it to the acupuncturist, he diagnosed cystitis during treatment. So for a while he treated me for cystitis as well as for the back. The cystitis cleared up fairly quickly. In the year since my last acupuncture treatment, I haven't had any problems with my back—not a twinge."

G.'s story exemplifies some truths about acupuncture.

- Acupuncture can be a satisfactory alternative to medication.
- In some cases acupuncture can prevent the need for surgery.
- If acupuncture works well for you in one condition, you are apt to respond well to treatment for a different condition.
- More than one problem can be treated by acupuncture at the same time.

✳

D., 59, is an artist, wife, and mother of grown children, who lives a physically active life in a remote part of coastal Maine. One year in June she made a routine trip alone by car to New York City.

"After three days in New York I got one of these hideous sinus headaches—completely incapacitating. I'd been going to a chiropractor, who manipulates things and keeps my spine straight. That's helped [her chronic sinus headaches] a lot, but I didn't know one in the city.

"A friend suggested acupuncture. I went right away, Thursday. I said I'd only be here till Sunday. The acupuncturist said, 'Okay, we're going to do one treatment a day, and I'm just going to concentrate on the neck.'

"She put all these needles around my face. On either side of my nose, right at the base, she put two needles with wires at the ends to which she attached an electrical pulsating thing. You feel sort of . . . ting! ting! ting! She put some needles in my hands. After twenty minutes or so, she sat me in a chair, tilted my head forward, and put some needles in the back of my neck.

"Right away I felt *somewhat* relieved, but you know you don't take these things away immediately. Within an hour after I left the office I could feel more relief. I took a bath and slept a while. I really woke up a new human being! I mean, I was able to eat a decent supper, and go to bed and sleep like a log, which I hadn't done for two nights. Unbelievable!

"I went back Friday for another treatment, and again on Saturday. In each treatment she increased the impulse to the needles at the base of my nose, so it got stronger and stronger. The acupuncturist said, 'We've got sort of a rush job here to get you going in three days.' She said ordinarily you do seven or eight, maybe ten treatments for sinus like mine.

"Saturday, after the third treatment, I was able to drive across town and pick up friends, go all the way out to Riverdale to a wedding and reception—the whole business—and back to town again without a problem. Normally, with a sinus crisis, I could never have done it.

"This sort of headache usually lasts three days. That's three days of trying everything—standing on my head, hot water bottles, going off every bit of food except a little gingerale and a baked potato. It upsets your stomach so you can't eat, you don't want to speak to anybody, you just want to bury your head. I sometimes get migraines—possibly stress-related, I've had them much less as time goes on. I can usually deter a migraine, which starts with visual disturbance, if I take an aspirin, lie down with my eyes covered, and just give up for a while. But I have *no* control over sinus headache—it gets right down into the bones under your eyes, and down into your teeth, and you get all this awful mucus.

"The acupuncturist in New York said I should have more treatment, but she didn't know anyone practicing in Maine. At my friend's house in Portland we went through the Yellow Pages."

This telephone directory showed an acupuncturist practicing about 70 miles from D.'s home, in partnership with a physician who was also trained in acupuncture. D. went for consultation, felt confidence in the acupuncturist, and was treated. During the next three weeks she returned twice a week for treatment. The four-hour round trip—only a few of the 70 miles are highway—meant that for those three weeks D. had to organize her life around the acupuncture schedule.

"We discussed some other problems I have—a bit of arthritis in my neck I've had off and on for about thirty years. And my left arm, it tightens up and the elbow hurts. She worked on that, and down my legs, all the way to the feet. I'd sometimes have fifteen needles in my face, and some into the scalp. Sometimes she'd roll me over onto my side, and put needles around the left shoulder particularly, and up the back and then down that whole left side.

"The only place that ever got sore was that spot between your forefinger and thumb. Each time—that was standard—she'd put a needle there and it got a little black and blue. Once she was upset because on my cheekbone there was a tiny bit of bleeding. It caused a small bruise. It didn't bother me, didn't hurt, and just faded right away. She was worried because she thought I might be bothered by it, but I wasn't.

"Sometimes when a needle was put in I'd say 'Ouch!'. I mean, it's not totally painless. But the pain goes right away.

"Both acupuncturists say there's no conflict between acupuncture and other kinds of medicine. I've continued seeing the chiropractor about once a month, because he has straightened my spine so much. After all those years of standing badly you have to keep at it, it's like exercise. In six months since my last acupuncture treatment, I've only had one sinus headache, and it lasted only a couple of hours.

"This acupuncturist in Maine said it's very curious that sometimes treatment can have quite dramatic effects, and sometimes the effects come quite a long while after treatment.

"The friend who first suggested acupuncture said, 'Now, don't expect miracles', but of course my experience was practically a miracle. The three treatments in New York made it possible for me to do the things I had to do. And the seven treatments up here—I felt better after each one. It was gradual, but cumulative. It's been a very positive experience. I'd go for some other problem, if there's any pain involved, at the drop of a hat. And I'd recommend acupuncture highly to anybody else, family as well as friends."

D.'s story shows some other things to remember about acupuncture.

 • There are some experienced acupuncturists practicing in rural areas.
 • For some conditions, the acute stage can be adequately relieved, but extensive treatment is needed to subdue chronic problems.

✳

When H. was about 60 she sought acupuncture treatment for pain radiating into her fingers, which she says came from pinched neck nerves.

"About seven years ago I went to a Chinese physician-acupuncturist and his acupuncture relieved me of the numbness and pain in my fingers for a period of at least a year, perhaps longer.

"I live in such intense pain that I'm not frightened of anything that might relieve me. As a matter of fact, acupuncture wasn't painful. Unpleasant, a little bit. With the electric machine hooked up to the needle, you feel little shocks, but nothing too frightening. With this doctor I had about ten treatments."

Five years later H. tried acupuncture again with a different practitioner.

"I went for about four weeks to a Korean, but I simply had no confidence. This one I dropped.

"Then I went to an American lady doctor who took up acupuncture after a lifetime in a Western medical specialty. She learned it from a Chinese acupuncturist. I had a series of sixteen treatments. It helped a little. But it didn't help much—after each treatment the pain would move from one area into another, and that discouraged me.

"I would say that it had not been very effective treatment for me in the long run. But I think that has to do with the condition I suffer from, which is going from bad to worse. With me it's a question of deteriorating disks and consequently also deteriorating nerve ends. I had reached, I believe, the end of my nerves' ends! They have become numb. I do not believe that at this stage of my condition acupuncture can help me anymore.

"But I do think it can alleviate the pain for a great length of time. I do believe in it very strongly. A friend of mine suffered from migraines all his life, and he was relieved by acupuncture."

H.'s story illustrates various aspects of acupuncture.

- Even though H. had suffered pain for a long time, her first treatment series produced relief which lasted over a year.
- H. mentions deteriorating disks. Acupuncture cannot repair structural defects.
- Acupuncture is not magic. You can believe

in it and have inadequate results, just as you can be skeptical about it and have good results.

✳

V., in his late 40s, is a partner in a New York accounting firm.

"I really hate novocaine," he says. "It seems like about seventeen hours of having it in your system. My dentist uses acupuncture. He tells you to cough, and when you do, he inserts the needle. Sometimes the needle is attached to the electro-pulsating machine. Sometimes the dentist twirls the needle manually.

"He's used acupuncture on me for filling cavities and for root-canal work. I didn't feel any pain at all. None!

"I certainly would try acupuncture for other problems besides dental work." V. grinned. "I'm completely in love with it!"

✳   ✳   ✳

Variables Which Affect Response to Treatment

Sometimes after a first, second or third treatment the problem for which you are being treated intensifies.

Acupuncture acts to coördinate physiological processes: needles stimulate activities of body chemistry so that various processes can take place compatibly. As your ailment developed, your system assumed the habit of functioning in one way. The counter-effect occurs when your system attempts to reject the stimulus directing it to function another way. However, after a short period of time the body gets used to the stimulus and starts working with it.

About 5% of acupuncture patients experience this counter-effect. You should not *expect* it to occur or, if it does, to last. There is no recorded instance of allergy to acupuncture.

Acute conditions often respond quickly. Muscle spasm pain can decrease significantly after one treatment; but it may take six or seven treatments to completely eliminate the consequences of, for example, having twisted your back. The sooner acupuncture treatment begins after onset of a health problem, the more rapidly you will respond.

Sometimes, as in D.'s story, a patient feels relief after the first treatment of a chronic complaint. Typically, this relief does not mean that one treatment is sufficient.

People usually put up with chronic pain for months or even years before resorting to acupuncture. Long-term pain makes you stand, sit, lie and move in ways that accommodate it. These distortions of normal posture produce tension which causes aches, cramps, spasms and even permanent musculoskeletal changes in parts of the body not obviously connected to the source of pain. When you do finally try acupuncture, don't expect instant results. You *can* expect steady decrease of pain. If you come to acupuncture after long use of drugs with annoying side effects, you can expect drug induced symptoms to disappear slowly.

The longer you've had a chronic problem, the more stubbornly will it resist treatment. If you've lived for years with a pattern of migraines, *tic douloureux* or sinus headaches, acupuncture needs time to change the pattern. Medication and surgery aren't instant magic; neither is acupuncture.

Previous unsuccessful remedies leave their mark on your system and can slow down, or even prevent, good response to acupuncture. Over time you've tried and been disappointed by other therapies. You should assume it will take time for acupuncture to prove its value to you.

Your age and general health affect the outcome of treatment. A woman of 21 strained her lower back on a summer job, stacking bales of hay. Sitting through college classes became agonizing. The pain on one side was gone after her first acupuncture treatment; she was completely relieved after the fourth. She learned to be careful of her back in bending and lifting—bending her knees instead of leaning over from the waist. She has maintained a high level of physical activity—working out at a gym, horseback riding, and karate training—with no back problems in the year since her last treatment.

Her mother, a woman of 53, experienced the same kind of strain while carrying groceries. The pain disappeared after five acupuncture treatments; but about six weeks later she felt the onset of sciatica, a common consequence of back injury. The sciatic nerve symptoms were completely relieved after four treatments.

The injuries were similar in location and degree; but the older woman needed more treatment to be completely rid of the resulting pain.

You get the most out of treatment if you follow instructions such as—for arthritis—keeping warm; for systemic lupus erythematosus, avoiding late night dissipation and exposure to sunshine; or—for cosmetic acupuncture—avoiding or limiting liquor and smoking. Just because instructions are simple, don't assume they're unimportant.

What Degree of Relief Is Satisfactory?

What we all want from any therapy is complete relief of the problem by quick painless methods. Short of this ideal, acceptable levels of satisfaction vary.

A violinist who develops tennis elbow—a painful condition described as self-limiting and seldom lasting more than a year—needs more thorough relief than a banker. Both people resent the pain; but the violinist needs a healthy elbow to earn a living and the banker doesn't.

L., 56, works "eight days a week" at his boat repair and marine salvage business in a Massachusetts fishing port. His face looks too young for his white hair. He is sturdy and muscular; physical strength is essential to his livelihood.

L.'s gallbladder was removed in 1975. Subsequently he complained of a protuberance developing in his upper diaphragm. Doctors suggested the problem was caused by the scar. They insisted the protuberance "was all in my head." L. suffered also from adhesions which affected his posture. In 1979 an operation was scheduled. Before the operation, L. took a surgical marker and drew a line with arrows pointing to it. "While you're in there, you check that place," he said.

The surgeon dealt with the adhesions, then explored the area his stubborn patient had marked. He removed a bony growth the size and shape of a small pinecone, with spines. It was in no way connected to any skeletal structure. It was certainly no product of L.'s imagination.

In 1981 and 1982 L. was operated on again for removal of bony growths in the same area. One is the size of an average woman's fist; the more recently-removed is smaller. After each operation L. felt little discomfort at the incision site; but had acute pain in his lower back and down his right leg to the top of his foot.

This severe, lasting pain was a gross impediment to L.'s work. One doctor suggested 6 weeks' bed rest. L. had to continue his physically demanding work. He managed by taking 16 to 18 Anacin and 6 Percocet (Percodam with Tylenol) daily. "I was scalloping and those dredges are heavy. Swallowing fistfuls of pills, and I don't like taking pills."

The severe back pain, with no obvious cause, continued. Doctors said they couldn't do anything for him, and suggested chiropractic treatment. Exercise and adjustments produced little improvement. The chiropractor suggested acupuncture.

"Well, I told him I hate needles. I'd had enough needles, with all those operations and tests. But I went.

"Those needles, they're like a thread. They're so thin he has to use a little brass tube, or they'd bend when he starts putting them in. He sets the tube and just taps the end, then removes the tube and moves the needle around to get it in just the right place. If it's not at the right place, it doesn't do any good.

"That first time he put needles around my stomach, around the incision, then all the way down my leg to my foot. Then he attached these electrodes, one at the top, one at the bottom. When he turned the rheostat on this little box I felt pain, like the one I'd been having [L. was not in pain crisis at the time of treatment] really moving all the way down my leg. He explained there's a connection between the meridian and the stomach and back."

L. felt some improvement after the first treatment, and had two more weekly treatments in this original series. Since then, whenever sporadic back pain hits, L. gets acupuncture treatment.

"It's the only thing that works for that back and leg pain. But I found if I had treatment in the morning I'd be no good for the rest of the day—too relaxed! Two weeks ago, my most recent treatment, I was feeling kind of pressed, people wanting this and that in a hurry. I felt edgy. That was the first time I was sensitive to the needles. After treatment the edgy feeling was gone."

Diagnosed as having osteoporosis, L. has been taking calcium pills for a year. He suspects a connection between osteoporosis and the bony growths. "Now it's been two years since the last growth was removed. Maybe it's slowing down."

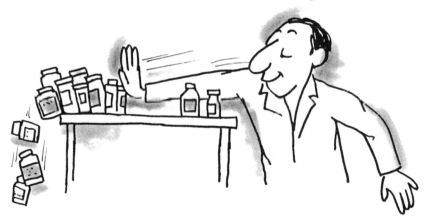

L. also takes 2 Motrin (400 mg.) daily. Standard dosage is 4 to 6. He no longer takes Anacin and Percocet. He is pleased by the reduction in medication.

L. works outdoors with heavy equipment in rough weather at all seasons. Traumas and musculoskeletal injuries are occupational hazards. With his complex and unusual medical history, L. will always be subject to pain episodes. However, by combining acupuncture treatment with as little medication as possible, L. is satisfied that he can maintain his "eight days a week" workload and still enjoy life with his wife and two young children.

✳

Since our bodies, lives and 'health fingerprints' vary widely, levels of satisfaction received from acupuncture treatment are subjective, not standard. Someone who has lived for a long time with chronic indigestion which fluctuates in intensity will find 45% improvement is really great relief.

If a tendency to gain weight is the bane of your existence, it is comforting to know that acupuncture helps fight weight-creep. Being treated for this problem every couple of years is a small price to pay for knowing you are not doomed forever to see food as the beloved enemy.

Cosmetic acupuncture requires many treatments and, to maintain results, refresher courses. Results in most cases are noticeable, but not as dramatic as with surgical facelifts. For some people this gentler modification of time's handiwork is preferable.

Only *you* know your acceptable level of satisfaction. Only *you* can judge how acupuncture results compare with other treatment you've had.

FOUR

Acupuncture For Weight Control and Smoking; Cosmetic Acupuncture

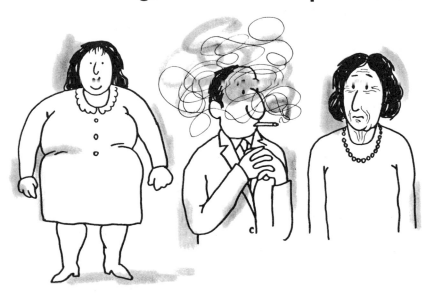

WITHOUT being hugely overweight, many of us must be eternally vigilant against weight-creep. Relax our guard, and suddenly the scales show an extra pound. Day after day that extra pound persists. Then it's two, and five. When fifteen pounds have crept under your skin, you can still get into most of your clothes, but the fleshy padding makes for a tight fit. In a few months there are more unwearable clothes in the closet than you want to think about. But you tell yourself you don't *look fat* in your new, next-size-up slacks. The pounds continue to creep aboard. One day, passing a shop window, you catch sight of a thick but familiar looking person—horrors! It's you!

For some people losing weight is simple. They muster determination, eat smaller portions of a wide variety of foods, lose weight slowly and maintain the desired lower weight. If you are such a fortunate person, skip this section.

More people resemble the brilliant journalist in her mid-forties who said, "I'm like an accordian. The minute I stop paying attention to eating carefully—which always seems to mean saying 'no' to things I really like—my waist, arms, neck and thighs bulge right out."

We accumulate unwanted pounds for different reasons: temperament, emotions, body chemistry, and the lives we lead contribute to the problem. Whatever your reason for wanting to lose weight, the question is not *what* to do, but how to live with the stunningly simple formula for weight loss: eat less, exercise more.

Some 40 million Americans struggle against fat. A $10 billion per year weight-loss service industry feeds on the people in this country who find dieting miserable and difficult. Depending on disposition and ability to pay, the desperate dieter has a multitude of approaches to choose from. Diet books; weight-loss centers; luxurious resorts where French chefs pamper the palate to ease you through a period of low-calorie meals; pre-measured frozen meals; nutrition formulas; surgical removal of fat; and over the counter medications, etc., all promise salvation when the Great Enemy, appetite, defeats willpower. This substantial industry indulges our natural desire to solve problems quickly and painlessly. If you have a history of dieting, and are once more trying to lose fifteen or twenty pounds, you know there's no free lunch.

Losing the weight is like armed revolution: arduous, but you feel triumphant when you achieve your goal. Now, you have to govern the country. Did the armed struggle phase teach you to eat a wide variety of foods in small portions? Did you form the habit of exercising more than your fat self ever did? If not, weight creep will begin to retake the territory. Many of us need help to lose weight. In picking your help, remember the old saying about get-rich-quick schemes: "If it sounds too good to be true, it probably is."

Acupuncture treatment for weight loss is *not* magic.

The acupuncture effect works gently, not dramatically, to reduce appetite, stimulate digestive processes, and give a sense of well-being and useful energy. Acupuncture can ease you into feeling satisfied after smaller meals, and stiffen your resistance to snacks and nibbles.

One woman said she first noticed the acupuncture effect halfway through a meal near the end of her first week of treatment. As she lifted a forkful of veal stew, she felt as if something in her abdomen shut down gently. She simply did not want that mouthful. She paid attention to the feeling and stopped eating, even though the food was delicious and she could have pushed herself to swallow more. At subsequent meals she began to take half her usual portion as a first serving. Soon she found she no longer wanted the other half as a second helping.

A man in his late thirties who had been a plump child, and as an adult suffered from weight-creep, said that acupuncture let him enjoy a normal relationship to food for the first time in his life. He was hungry at mealtimes, but found he could enjoy good food without craving the extra kick of extra helpings.

Acupuncturists use different techniques for weight management, either regular needles at appropriate body, leg and arm points; or ear acupuncture.

In ear acupuncture, points on the external ear are stimulated to calm or tonify the stomach, digestion and metabolism. Methods of stimulation include surgical steel staples; sutures, either removable or soluble; metal pellets taped over the points; or, most commonly, several press needles with flat circular handles and points about 1/8 inch long.

After swabbing your ear thoroughly with alchohol, the acupuncturist presses each needle in firmly. It can hurt, but not much, and not for more than a few minutes. One point is usually more sensitive than the others. Each needle is covered with surgical tape. One acupuncturist tells you to press the needles at least seven times a day; and whenever you feel hungry or are tempted to snack. You will also be told to keep the needled ear dry. If tape gets wet it loses sticking power. Loose tape does not protect pierced skin from infection, or needles from falling out or, worse, tumbling into the ear canal—a remote possibility, but one of which you should be aware.

Needles are left in for a week, after which they are removed, and fresh needles placed in the other ear. The number of treatments depends on individual response to acupuncture and on how much you want to lose.

Obviously you'll have to wash your hair while in treatment. Fold a dry washcloth into a pad which just covers your ear. Hold it against the needled ear and shampoo with the other hand. It's a bit awkward, but manageable.

Some people experience a slight increase in appetite during the first week of ear acupuncture. Don't be discouraged if this happens to you—it's a temporary result of metabolic adjustment to the stimulus of acupuncture. Pretty soon—in most cases, early in the second week—your appetite shrinks so that you become comfortable eating less than you used to before starting treatment.

Make sure to select your smaller-portion meals from the four basic food categories: dairy; meats, dried beans, poultry and fish; fruits and vegetables; breads and cereals. Since 1977 there has been serious revision of what kinds and proportions of basic food groups make a healthy diet, with emphasis on reducing percentage of protein intake. You may have special needs: a vegetarian will want to select necessary proteins from non-meat sources; post-menopausal women need more calcium than when they were younger, to mention just two examples.

If you don't usually exercise, start; if you do, add some vigorous moves to your routine. Exercise not only works off calories, it helps cut your appetite by stimulating production of the body's natural tranquillizers, beta-endorphins. Try to exercise about an hour before eating.

One man said acupuncture was no good. He found himself pressing the ear needles with one hand as he ate a double-scoop ice cream cone from the other. Acupuncture could obviously do no more for him than all the other diet aids he had tried during the last twenty years—including a hospital obesity clinic.

In our war against weight-creep, psychological factors are as important as physiological ones. Don't fight the benign effects of acupuncture by expecting the needles to do the whole job for you: they are not magic wands! Form the habit of listening to your body. Acupuncture dulls the edge of appetite. You feel satisfied earlier in the meal than you used to. Pay attention to your response—it's the difference between having a radio on for background noise, and really listening to the music.

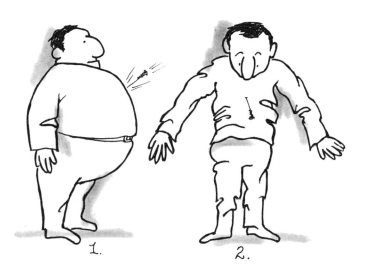

By nature you may be a rapid eater. Learn to make food consumption last at least twenty-minutes. Use a kitchen timer at breakfast to get a feeling for how long this is. You can learn to stretch out the pleasure of eating, whether you lunch alone or dine surrounded by friends and family who seem to be able to eat all they want without getting fat. Forget what your mother said—there is no virtue in a clean plate. In restaurants, or other people's houses, remind yourself that it's better for you to let food go *to waste* than *to waist*. You're spending money, enduring a little pain, and being faithful about pressing the needles. Why override the effects of treatment by eating fast, or having another bite when you're satisfied?

Expect to lose weight gradually, from 2 to 5 pounds a week, depending on the amount of excess weight you've been carrying. Slow, steady weight loss is better for your system and your skin than a dramatic decrease.

You reach your goal and the needles are removed. What's to keep the weight off, now that you're no longer having treatment?

An important factor is that you've been eating realistically during treatment. Your diet consisted of eating *less,* not of eating a narrowly restricted range of foods; or of living on nutrition formulas. End of treatment does not mean the end of gastronomic austerity from which the average dieter emerges with a rebellious craving for chocolate cake. You haven't been in dieters' isolation— your senses aren't starved for something which tastes good, as a relief from weeks of limited flavors.

In many people, decreased appetite and a definite sense of well-being persist for months after the ear acupuncture needles have been removed. These lingering effects are another factor which supports you in maintaining weight loss.

Since acupuncture is a drug free method of controlling weight, you can feel safe about returning for further treatment if, after months or years, the old troublesome excess appetite returns. It's a great relief to know that you can fight off weight-creep without having to be heroic!

✳   ✳   ✳

Ear acupuncture is also used to help people stop smoking. Because many smokers are afraid of gaining weight as a penalty for giving up cigarettes, some acupuncturists treat for both problems together; the necessary acupuncture effects are compatible.

A heavy smoker—smoking a pack or more a day—is addicted to nicotine. Addiction is a word we generally associate with junkies and street crime. It may seem harsh to use the word in connection with cigarette smoking, but the label is accurate.

Addiction in this case means that your system has adapted neurochemically to a regular level of response to nicotine. When the level drops a process of adjustment takes place, involving biochemical changes which produce disagreeable signs and symptoms of withdrawal. Many smokers complain that quitting brings on excess mucus, sore throat, headache and chest pains; along with mood changes and restlessness. This withdrawal syndrome can last for weeks after the cigarette you swore would be your last.

Acupuncture works on the autonomic nervous system to prevent signs and symptoms of withdrawal. It controls physical signs; calms restlessness; and alleviates the anxiety and sense of deprivation aroused by giving up smoking.

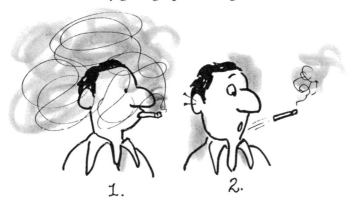

1.   2.

Acupuncture helps you accomplish your goal by reinforcing your willpower. However, just as in treatment for weight loss, you must understand that the needles cannot do the whole job for you.

One chainsmoking woman in her late fifties sought acupuncture treatment to break her habit. The acupuncturist told her that acupuncture would cut her consumption in half the first week, and in half again each week until she was smoking so few cigarettes that she would be able to give them up relatively easily. After the third treatment the woman was down to five cigarettes a day; after the fourth she stopped smoking. She planned to have one more treatment to reinforce her new non-smoking condition. But suddenly she had to go to another city to attend the death and funeral of a close relative whom she loved deeply. Her lifelong response to stress had been to smoke more cigarettes than usual. Overwhelmed by agonizing circumstances she resumed smoking, even though for some time she found the process disagreeable. Other factors in her life overrode the acupuncture effect.

❋

P., 35, is a writer who for many years smoked over two packs daily.

"For quite a while I'd wanted to quit smoking. I'd been leading up to it by taking up running and tennis again. For a long time I didn't get much exercise, but over the last year and a half I was trying to get back into shape, so smoking loomed as more and more of a conflict.

"The problem was I could imagine myself in any situation without smoking cigarettes, if necessary; but I just couldn't picture working without them. But it got to the point where I felt I had to quit. I would risk never writing another word rather than feel as awful as I did when I finished writing and saw a full ashtray. I really didn't know which way to turn. I didn't want to screw it up by making any more botched cold-turkey attempts."

P. called the American Cancer Society to ask what choices there were if he wanted help to stop smoking. One recommendation was acupuncture.

"I thought if I do it with acupuncture I'm going to have to pay for it, and it's under somebody else's authority, I'll feel like I'm on a team. So I went to an acupuncturist . . he was Chinese, and an M.D. as well.

"He took my blood pressure. He asked what I did for a living, and a couple of relevant questions. I didn't feel he was very interested in my answers. He gave me some clippings to read about his acupuncture treatment. He told me to give him my cigarettes which I had in my top pocket. I did, and he very efficiently tore them up and threw them out. I thought that was very good. He also showed me a picture of a diseased lung. I looked at it and sort of shrugged and said, 'big deal.' It really didn't impress me too much.

"I sat on a bench and he rubbed my ears with alchohol. He took these two flat circular little pins and shoved them in just in front of the protrusion at the front part of the ear. It must have been into cartilage, because there was sort of a crunch. He put one on each side and covered it with tape.

"Then he gave me the basic facts and figures: you're not to smoke, you come back once a week for the next four weeks, and at the end of that time you'll be fine. If you ever relapse, get back here as soon as you can, we'll do the treatment again.

"He said the quit ratio was high, but the rate of recidivisim is fairly high too, for reasons which I didn't quite understand. He said if I had an urge to smoke I should rub the needles in a circular motion. He explained the theory behind it, that it was cutting off certain nerves and blocking the appetite for cigarettes. If the needles fell out, I could come back. He was pretty thorough about telling me what to do.

"Well, I left and ran to the corner and bought a pack of cigarettes and immediately smoked two of them.

"I don't have a whole lot of faith in doctors; and I felt this acupuncturist was another case of a professional who didn't give me much feeling of warmth or sympathy. I'm not sure a doctor's supposed to give you that, actually . . . When I left the office I sort of resented how quickly it had all happened: I was in and out in about half an hour. I think that's one reason I immediately went and smoked. Another probably is that I had a tennis match in a tournament that afternoon. I hadn't known about it when I made the acupuncture appointment.

"This was a period I'd managed to set aside to come to grips with my smoking problem. I'd already made a week's worth of effort to quit cold-turkey. I'd told myself it's now or never. If it meant leaving every morning and playing tennis all day and having a good time and eating out every night, I'd do it. I'd kind of built a small vacation around this idea of quitting smoking.

"So there I was on the street with a new pack of cigarettes! I played my match. Lost. Went home. I guess I had one
cigarette that evening. Then I threw the pack away. Said, 'I'm not
going to smoke.' I haven't had a cigarette since. That was seven
months ago.

"It was really no problem sticking to that resolve. I
don't feel the acupuncture eliminated my desire to smoke. I think
what it did eliminate—and this is where it really helped—was
some kind of anxiety and extreme nervousness that I used to feel
when I denied myself cigarettes. I had the urge to smoke; but
fighting the urge, I seemed to be in a clear, calm state. I felt like
nothing could bother me. On the other hand, I didn't want to do
anything, either.

"I don't know to what degree that was biologically or
psychologically created by the acupuncture; or to what degree it
was due to having a period of time in which absolutely the only
thing I wanted to think about was quitting smoking. I let everything else go. I don't want to overdramatize, but it was such an
effort, in a quiet way, that every minute without smoking was like
a tremendously successful experience in life. Just the fact that I was
able to breathe and walk around and talk to people and read and
eat, and not smoke at any of those times was like doing a great
piece of work.

"At the second treatment he took the needles out and
put others in the same places. He asked how I was doing. I
immediately confessed my sins. But by then, after a week, I'd
found that with each day my resolve and determination got
stronger. By the second session I was pretty firmly committed to
not smoking. It would have taken a catastrophe to make me smoke
again. The acupuncturist, in his way, was pretty supportive. He
reminded me strongly not to lapse, and said I'd find it gets easier
by the day.

"At the beginning I was told it's usually a five-treatment
program. He charged $40 a treatment. A friend asked why I didn't
quit after the second treatment, since I was doing so well. The

thing is, I wanted to be sure the job would be done. I guess I'm the kind of person who figures, well, I signed up for the program, I've got to go through with it. He said five treatments, so that's what I had. I certainly didn't feel he was pressuring me to have any more than that. He said some people have a cigarette now and then in the first week after they finish treatment. Maybe he said that to take the pressure off, when you know you've had the last treatment.

"I would go for acupuncture treatment for anything I felt warranted it. Other things besides smoking. And I'd certainly recommend it to friends—without thinking twice."

Acupuncture for Face Treatment

Your reasons for wanting to do something about your face may be professional, personal or a combination of both. Men and women alike worry about how prospective employers see them, especially when making mid-life career changes. A woman who returns to outside work after years of paying dues to family life is particularly vulnerable. She worries that her face gives the wrong impression of her real vigor and capacity for hard work. How you look on camera, at Board meetings or in public life can affect your self assurance and ability to perform well. You may have kept your body in shape by diet and exercise, and feel that the face you see in the mirror has aged more than the rest of you. Should you have a few surgical tucks—a facelift?

What kind of change are you looking for? Acupuncture face treatment is *not* a substitute for plastic surgery. The procedure does not change facial structures; it will not remove heavy under-eye bags and deeply sagging jowls. Obviously, if you want a new nose, mouth or chin, you should investigate the possibilities of plastic and reconstructive surgery. What acupuncture can do is give your face a less worn look so that you present a fresher, brighter appearance to yourself in the mirror, and to the world. One woman in her mid-sixties said, "I can't really measure the difference, but my dentist who hadn't seen me for three months asked me the other day what I'd been doing to my face—it looked younger and healthier."

Faces show wear and tear differently. If you have light dry skin, your face will show the ravages of summer sun-worshipping as early as your mid-thirties. Slightly oily olive-toned complexions are more durable. However, as years pass, even people who tanned beautifully in youth start looking grey and blotchy when their tans fade. The sun's ultraviolet rays thicken the outer layer of skin, and break down substances in the dermis, or inner layer, which make skin elastic. No matter how dark your skin, it can be damaged by too much sun.

Other factors affect your skin, like demands of work, and the climate you live in, matters over which you have no control. Heavy dissipation, lack of sleep and poor nutrition also leave their marks on your face.

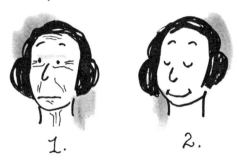

1.   2.

Acupuncture face treatment stimulates facial nerves whose action improves muscle tone. Needles are placed in wrinkles and lines. Patients say facial needles don't hurt, although you may feel a light prickling here and there. Needles are also placed in leg and hand points to stimulate the digestive system, and to relax you so that circulation of blood and energy is improved. Low-level electro-pulsing is applied to some needles. A light facial massage follows needle treatment.

Acupuncture face treatment affects your general system, even though treatment emphasis is on the face; therefore you can expect some of the same responses that follow treatment for other conditions: improved energy, and a heightened sense of well-being.

12 to 15 sessions are usual for a first series of face treatments. After that, occasional treatments keep your facial nerves, muscles and skin toned up. In considering acupuncture face treatment, think also about protecting your investment by limiting exposure to sun, tobacco and alcohol. Once again, acupuncture can do a lot for you, but it can't do the whole job!

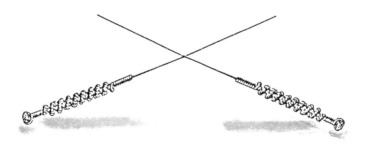

FIVE

Acupuncture and Substance Abuse

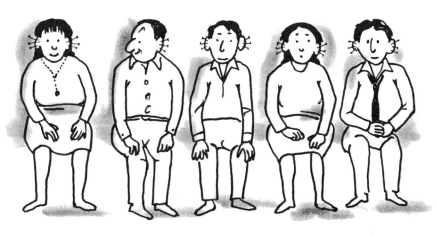

YOU know you have a problem. The good highs were so long ago they might as well have been someone else's. Now, the drink or the pills or the dope mostly just take the edge off feeling bad. You think a lot about keeping supplies handy, because time just doesn't move at all when you're waiting to get that dose of whatever substance—to dissolve anxiety and tension, at least for a while. Miss your dose, and all you can think about is how awful you feel.

People talk in different ways about the stuff that controls their lives. "My eyes look like two oysters in a bucket of blood. Must have been the eighth Scotch last night. A Bullshot'll do the trick—hair of the dog." "Behind a hundred dollar jones, man, it's pure misery waitin' to take care of business, get straight." "It was nothing more than usual. But around two a.m. when I got home, my heart started going like a jackhammer. Swear, I thought I was dying. Now I'm careful, just do a couple of lines before the first set. No problem." "I don't *need* Valium, just take one before staff meetings. Or when my job gives me the blues." "You can skin-pop heroin and not get hooked." "Pot's no big deal—just like having a beer." "I never drink before noon." "I do coke, but only on weekends." "Sure I'd like to quit. But the stuff won't let me go."

Circumstances, chemicals of choice, and styles of substance abuse differ; but addictive behavior is remarkably similar at any social or economic level. If you're hooked, you tend to deny the existence or extent of the problem. You persist in a pleasureless state. And you accept the common myth that the drug, not the user, makes the addict, as if the substance had power and will of its own. Literature supports the myth: in *Othello* Shakespeare said, "O thou invisible spirit of wine! If thou hadst no name to be known by, let us call thee devil!" In the nineteenth century, three years before he died Thomas de Quincey wrote, "Thou hast the keys of Paradise, oh just, subtle and mighty opium!" United States Prohibitionists campaigned against "Demon Rum." With references to "King Heroin" and "Lady Snow," contemporary junkie poems personify drugs as if chemicals, like people, were capable of destructive intent.

You know that alcohol and other drugs have benign uses. It's the purpose for which you take them that makes the difference between *use* and *abuse*. Because your purpose in taking a substance is intricately linked to its effects on you—pain and problems fade away, life is more bearable—abuse leads to *dependency*. During the development of your dependency, complex physiological processes work to let your system adapt to the presence of chemicals.

Living with the regular presence of drugs in your body is possible because of our brilliant human capacity to adapt to environment, internal or external. An area of the brain which controls the function of internal organs and systems receives messages from neurotransmitters saying, "this substance throws things off balance, we have to make some adjustments." Physiological adjustments, expressing the human system's tendency toward internal balance, account for the decreasing effect of a specific amount of one drug taken by one method. To increase the effect you may take more, or take it by a different method; or modify one drug by combining it with another. But unless you kill yourself by overdosing, each time you vary the formula your marvelous physiology keeps right on making these minute adjustments to the new quantity or mix of chemicals; and defining the new input as 'normal.' To get high, you have to go beyond each newly defined 'normal' stage.

If your dose is delayed your system is abruptly deprived of the chemical to which it has learned to adapt. Neurotransmitters begin to send the brain messages saying, "help, we're running out of fuel" and the brain, in turn, transmits the information to organs and systems which react by producing the signs and symptoms of withdrawal. These can include pounding of the heart; pallor; wheezing cough; shaking; feeling cold and sweating at the same time; stomach cramps; dilated pupils; excess saliva which you have to keep swallowing; anxiety; tension; insomnia; aching bones; and a general sense of dread. The morning grumpiness typical of heavy drinkers is a consequence of the longest non-drinking period in twenty-four hours: after sleeping for seven to nine hours, you wake to the onset of withdrawal. Advanced alcoholics often wake up after three or four hours' sleep feeling anxious—in many cases, anxious enough to get up and have a drink before trying to get a little more sleep.

Long after you've abandoned all hope of re-experiencing the original pleasure the drug gave, you must feed your habit, or feel sick. This ancient predicament gave rise to the myth of drug-as-demon, a creature intent on keeping you in its clutches. The myth feeds on the real difficulties of getting clean and/or sober, and staying that way. But it's not the drug that refuses to let go of you; it's your well-adapted system which clings to the drug—after all, it has spent much energy learning to live with it.

Whatever method is used, effective treatment for substance abuse requires detoxification—getting the stuff out of your system; and a recovery program—specific, realistic plans for a life without your habit. It is arguable just how voluntarily anyone enters treatment. The decision to do so is usually forced by external events: you are threatened with losing your job; brought up short by a lover or spouse who refuses to live with you and your habit anymore; or get into trouble with the law, and the judge gives you a choice—program or penalty. In these circumstances your enthusiasm for detox and determination to persist in treatment are understandably limited.

For reasons linked to motivation and health, substitution therapy is standard treatment. The idea is to give you a drug with similar but not identical action to the one you've been using. Librium, for example, prevents convulsions when the heavy user stops drinking alcohol, which is a central nervous system depressant. Valium is often given to help you during detoxification from cocaine. Similarly, methadone and Darvon-N, among other drugs, are given for narcotics withdrawal. Ideally, the substitute drug is given in closely monitored decreasing dosage, retraining your system to define ever lower levels as 'normal' until you aren't taking any drug at all.

Unfortunately, as the history of opiate abuse in this country shows, while it may seem logical to use one drug against another, it doesn't always work. Morphine, derived from opium and superbly powerful against acute pain, at one time was used against opium addiction. During our Civil War morphine was not only given for combat injuries, but also dispensed liberally to cure dysentery, which could incapacitate soldiers. A severe social problem of the post-Civil War era was widespread morphine addiction, commonly known as "Soldiers' Disease." Heroin, synthesized from morphine, was initially considered non-addictive, and given to cure morphine addiction. In the body heroin quickly turns back into morphine. Heroin proved every bit as addictive as the morphine whose abuse it was intended to cure. In the late 1960s methadone looked like a winner in the fight against heroin addiction. But over the years evidence accumulated that methadone produces unhealthy side effects; worse, methadone itself became a drug of abuse, sold on the street just like heroin. . . Darvon-N, another synthetic painkiller used to treat people withdrawing from narcotics, carries with it the problem of any similar drug: tolerance develops quickly, and you can easily get hooked. We have yet to develop a painkiller that doesn't offer possibilities of addiction.

Experienced workers in the field of substance abuse generally agree that for any kind of treatment to succeed, it must be given along with a program that strengthens your ability to cope with social, practical and psychological problems related to addiction. In our culture social life regularly involves liquor and often includes drugs. It takes more determination to avoid these substances than to use them. And memory has a way of softening pain. Months and years after detoxification, when your health improves, when you no longer need your dose to stop hurting, it's tempting to think a little taste can't do any harm. People who once were addicted to heroin have said that even years after quitting they can recall every physical detail of the pleasure the drug once gave. Many non-drinking alcoholics live in a tense state that A.A. calls "white knuckle sobriety."

Acupuncture reduces the intensity of physical signs of withdrawal; stimulates the digestive system and other avenues of elimination, to rid the body of toxic wastes; and relieves depression and insomnia, which can last for a long time after detoxification, and really undermine your willpower. The nature of addiction suggests that in the long run drugless therapy is more enduringly effective than drug-assisted treatment. But responsible treatment focuses on the patient, not on proving that one therapeutic method is better than another in all cases. Medication can be given to help deal with pain in detoxification, so long as it is not the type of drug known to block the action of acupuncture. Recovering alcoholics struggling to stay sober during family crisis or on the first non-drinking vacation, can be given disulfiram (Antabuse) in dosage carefully tailored to the individual's general health. Antabuse is not a substitute for liquor: a truth-or-consequences drug, it produces red flushes, palpitations and vomiting if you take any alcohol while it's in your system. It is a tool to bridge rough times in recovery; and in many cases has been found compatible with ongoing acupuncture treatment.

Some acupuncturists in private practice treat people with substance abuse problems. A responsible practitioner will explain that treatment alone cannot do the whole job. Psychotherapy, and joining a 12-step group such as A.A. or Narcotics Anonymous, provide a support system which you must have to benefit from treatment. After all, most of your time is spent outside the treatment room. Out there, you need all the help you can get.

A substance abuse clinic provides a package deal that includes treatment along with phased, structured counseling and other practical resources. Dr. Michael Smith is the United States pioneer in designing clinics which incorporate Chinese medical principles of herbal and acupuncture treatment with in-house counseling and recommendation to attend A.A. or N.A. meetings. Many people who use acupuncture in substance abuse treatment were trained at Lincoln Center for Substance Abuse, where Dr. Smith is medical director. From Maine to California, acupuncturists interviewed for this chapter mentioned Dr. Smith's clinic as an important, influential model. In this instance, therefore, it seems foolish to maintain anonymity.

Lincoln Center for Substance Abuse occupies a building in the South Bronx a few blocks from Lincoln Hospital—a New York City hospital—with which it is affiliated. You enter a large room with forty-nine high-backed easy chairs ranged along the walls, and in short rows which fill most of the central space. The room is bright and gives a sense of friendly busyness. The social worker has his own office; but the six acupuncturists and three MD-acupuncturists tend their paperwork at a couple of long tables in full view of clients. Three-hundred-fifty people per day receive treatment; the file on each client is updated immediately after treatment. Most of the people sitting in the chairs have straight acupuncture needles dangling from their ears; a few also have needles in hands, arms, legs and feet. Six cubicles provide privacy for treatment which requires undressing.

The layout of the clinic may appear improvised; but it serves specific purposes. Open workspace allows staff members to consult each other as they record each client's progress. Nobody has to run to another room for a client's folder before treating, or to ask a colleague, who may have seen the client two days ago, for additional information. Many people feel anxious about treatment. This communal setting, where you see everybody else with needles in them, reduces stress. (Needle-fear is notable in people who used to shoot up drugs.) During treatment, you can talk to other clients and compare notes. Observing the ethnically diverse staff members interact with each other, and give treatment, you see them as human beings, not just impersonal experts. Clients are not urged to leave the minute needles are removed—some people prefer to sit and collect themselves for a while before going out. The atmosphere is casual and open, yet order prevails. There is none of the icy briskness so many of us associate with hospitals, where it seems that matters urgently important to you are settled by other people behind closed doors.

Lincoln's clients reflect the demographics of addiction: most are Hispanic or black, range in age from teens on up, and live in poverty. However, the clinic also treats people who can afford to fly to New York and stay for two weeks, travelling to the South Bronx from midtown by limousine.

Fees are on a sliding scale, from $28 to $7 per treatment. If you can't pay, you are helped to get a Medicaid card, which also entitles you to carfare to and from the clinic.. (State regulations about acupuncture, substance abuse treatment and Medicaid vary.)

When you enter the Lincoln program, you must expect to go daily for detoxification. Along with acupuncture, you are given teabags of an herbal mix to make a drink which is relaxing and cleansing, but neither sedative nor habit-forming. You can drink as much of this as you wish. You also receive written instructions; and descriptions of the process your body goes through in detoxification, and what these signs tell you about your health. Daily urine tests and breathalizer tests are given. After a few days you are assigned a counselor. Once the tests show your system is free of drugs and/or alcohol, you are assigned to a "clean group." Group work focuses on practical problem-solving and mutual therapeutic help.

Group work helps you deal with psychological and

social changes that occur when you stop taking the substance to which you are addicted. You may find your old buddies pretty boring if they're still using and you're not: drinking and drugs form the theme of an awful lot of talk among heavy users, who can spend hours comparing brands, sources and experiences of being high, mellow, strung out and wired. Walking a pal through an overdose; what they said I did in my blackout; the jerks who put me on a bad trip; and the night the Feds almost busted my dealer in the men's room. . . When you no longer share the action you lose your zest for these familiar war stories; but you may also feel nostalgic for the old days when you were part of the scene. New associates, and counseling, strengthen your drive to be clean/sober when, as often happens, your life requires spending time with people who still use what you have given up. Without a support system, detoxification can be a revolving door: with a clean system you could resume your habit and a low dosage would give you the effects you still crave.

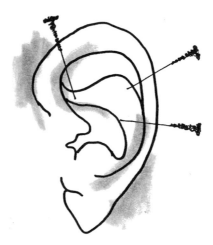

At first, whether your problem is alcohol or drugs, your acupuncture treatment is standard. The condition of addiction, and the signs and symptoms of withdrawal, dominate other patterns of disorder in your system. After detoxification, treatment is adjusted in accordance with your particular condition and constitution. For example, when palpitations, stomach cramps and nausea fade, you may notice a low-back problem which has been there all along, but obscured by other, more powerful miseries. This condition would then be treated by needling other points along with continued ear treatment for your addictive problem. As with acupuncture treatment generally, other health disorders may be treated at the same time as the primary one which brought you to the clinic.

In the course of treatment some people find they lose their taste for smoking cigarettes, or cut down, or quit, even though the habit hadn't worried them—it seemed minor compared to their drug/alcohol addiction.

Typically, alcoholics who stop drinking liquor take up massive coffee drinking. Coffee is warm and stimulating, and people usually sweeten it, compensating for the reduced sugar intake caused by being liquor-free. While coffee drinking is certainly not in the same category of problems as alcoholism, it seems to be a mild form of substitution therapy. People treated with acupuncture and herbs do not develop this boundless craving for coffee.

Another common change reported during acupuncture treatment for substance abuse has to do with food. Alcoholics find they can look at food without the familiar gag reflex. As time passes, clients often report, "You know, I feel much better if I eat _____." Generally the dietary change is for the better. In addiction you eat opportunistically, according to craving and convenience, without thinking about nutrition. As acupuncture stimulates your system toward health, fresh food becomes more appealing than junk food. At the clinic, this acupuncture-prompted tendency toward healthier eating is reinforced by nutritional advice.

The streets are full of people who went cold-turkey in prison, then came out and started building up their habits again. Expensive restaurants and country clubs are full of people who went to "health farms" or spas to dry out, then celebrated return to normal life with a couple of drinks. If you go to Lincoln, or

78

similar clinics, for treatment, you are not defended against temptation the way you would be in a residential therapeutic program.
Rich or poor, you'll still spend most of your time in the world
where you acquired your addiction. In the context of daily life the
innovative combination of methods used at Lincoln is astonish-
ingly successful.

Possibly other clinics using the combination of
acupuncture, herbs and conventional counseling methods, will
differ from Lincoln in ways which may be important to you. Some
clinics accept walk-in clients no matter what the addictive problem; others will not take alcoholics as walk-in clients, but will
accept drug abusers on this basis. Because of agreements with a
sponsoring hospital, a clinic might accept only inpatients of that
hospital; or outpatients already enrolled in a department of the
hospital.

RESOURCES

**Acupuncture
and
Substance Abuse**

Acupuncture Clinic
3245 Lorna Road
Birmingham, Alabama 01190
(205) 979-4079

Acupuncture Detox Center
1207 Mount, Missoula
Montana 59801
(406) 721-2147

Green Cross of the Americas
1510 U Street, N.W.
Washington, DC 20009
(202) 265-0100

Hennepin County Medical Center
Substance Abuse Clinic
701 Park Avenue South
Minneapolis, MN 55415
(612) 347-6111

Kings County Addictive Disease Hospital
66 Albany Avenue, Brooklyn, NY 11203
(718) 735-2856

Lincoln Center for Substance Abuse
349 East 140th Street, Bronx, NY 10454
(212) 993-3100

Somerville Acupuncture Center
77 Holland Street, Somerville
Massachusetts 02144
(617) 776-2020

Quan Yin Acupuncture & Herb Center
513 Valencia Street, San Francisco
California 94110
(415) 861-1101

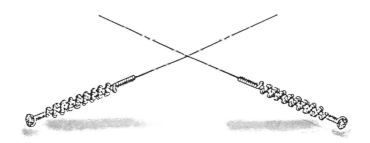

SIX

Choosing Your Acupuncturist; State Regulations; Health Insurance and Acupuncture

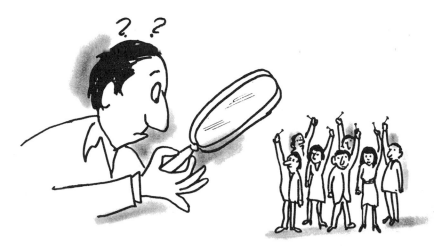

IN looking for an acupuncturist, try the obvious first: ask a person who knows one. Most of us do this at one time or other when looking for an accountant, dentist, doctor or lawyer. There are probably more people among your acquaintances and colleagues than you realize, who have had acupuncture treatment. Track down leads. Talk to the patient. Get a frank opinion of the practitioner. There's nothing like a firsthand account for dramatic clarity. What did this person get treatment for? How long had the problem lasted before treatment? How many treatments were needed? What did it cost? Would this person return to this acupuncturist?

Whatever you learn, remember that the condition for which your informant was treated may differ from yours, even if the complaints sound alike. Low-back pain, for example, is a catchall term for a misery which can affect five different people five different ways. No two bodies are exactly alike. After a few decades of wear and tear, the bodies of even identical twins differ in some ways.

The indefinable chemistry between practitioner and patient is not always transferable. You've probably had the experience of recommending someone's professional competence, only to have the person to whom you gave the referral say that so-and-so seems *competent* enough, but. . . Something was missing for effective collaboration.

A friend referred a woman with a back problem to "the best doctor in town for that kind of thing." The woman made an appointment, not realizing that acupuncture is the treatment for which this doctor is famous. The woman was asked to sign a release form which mentioned needles. She said she was afraid of needles, and did not want acupuncture; but signed anyway, so that she could have the treatment if she changed her mind. She talked to the doctor, found him very impressive, and had no trouble deciding to try acupuncture. Treatment involved needles in ankles and wrists, and up her legs. In recalling the experience she said that she was in such pain before the appointment that she could barely walk. After treatment she still hurt; but most of the pain was gone by the next day. Gradually it went away completely.

"In the last six years," she reported, "whenever I get a hint the pain might come back, I go for another treatment. I've also done body work to learn how to prevent lower back pain."

This is the only patient interviewed who was surprised into acupuncture. Clearly, she had no predisposition to believe this mode of treatment would help her, but it did.

If you can't track down a personal referral, get in touch with one of the organizations listed under RESOURCES, at the end of this chapter. If you live in a state without an acupuncture association, the association of a neighboring state may be helpful. The American Association of Acupuncture and Oriental Medicine (AAAOM) can provide a list of member acupuncturists in your region, as can the Center for Chinese Medicine, and the Traditional Acupuncture Institute. Such lists are not necessarily recommendations, simply a base of information for your own further inquiries.

Some physicians are happy to refer patients to acupuncture. It is nearly as frustrating to the doctor as it is painful and demoralizing for you, when one conventional remedy after another fails to improve your condition. A conservative internist surprised a patient by suggesting acupuncture for longlasting back pain of unknown origin. Some years before, the doctor had received successful acupuncture treatment for his own sore neck. He referred the patient to the same licensed (non-MD) acupuncturist. With luck, you will find a doctor who knows about acupuncture and has observed treatment by a qualified acupuncturist.

There are two kinds of physician-acupuncturists. One is the MD who has had thorough acupuncture training; who may even have practiced as an acupuncturist before becoming an MD; and who uses acupuncture routinely in treating patients. The other is the MD with a certificate for completing an acupuncture course for Medical Act licensees. In New York, the standard for such courses is 300 hours' training. Some physicians have given time to the study of acupuncture in order to provide this option for patients; or, in other cases, because they live in remote areas and acupuncture allows them to relieve pain without drugs.

In both conventional medicine and acupuncture the practitioner's art develops and becomes richer with experience. A well-trained experienced acupuncturist has concentrated on this health-care method, and uses it exclusively in treating patients. A conventional MD with a short course of acupuncture training cannot know the subject as well. Both conventional medicine and acupuncture demand a sound knowledge of anatomy and pathology; but acupuncturists are trained to view physiology—the functioning processes of the body—differently from the way Western medicine sees it. People with real competence in both acupuncture and conventional medicine do exist; but they are exceptional.

Depending on where you live, medical referral may be your only route to acupuncture treatment. There are still some doctors who, when you ask about acupuncture, react as if you'd suggested spraying your sciatic nerve with the blood of a black rooster. People have been discouraged from trying acupuncture because a doctor made them feel foolish for asking about it. This attitide is beginning to disappear, but patients still meet it once in a while. To bolster your confidence in pursuing your search, remember the good teacher's slogan: there are no stupid questions.

✳ ✳ ✳

Americans have been finding their way into acupuncture since post-Revolutionary times; but establishment of United States schools for formal acupuncture training was a development of the late 1960s. Before there were schools, Americans who wanted to become acupuncturists had to find training in U.S. Chinese communities; or travel to Asia, Canada or Europe. Some correspondence schools, serving farflung acupuncture students, arranged supervised practical work upon completion of studies. At present most acupuncture schools are residential: classroom attendance is mandatory. The standard toward which most schools are moving, if they are not already there, is a 2-year basic acupuncture course, about 1,000 hours of lectures, demonstrations and practical work; followed by a period of supervised clinical internship. In addition to topics special to acupuncture, students must take between 20 and 30 credits of college-level science: anatomy, physiology, pathology, chemistry and biology. Some schools also require credits in social sciences: psychology, anthropology or sociology. Generally at least 2 years of college, or a bachelor's degree, or work experience in a health profession are required for admission. The commitment in time and work demanded by leading acupuncture schools is similar to a university graduate program. Schools also offer advanced work in acupuncture specialties; and sessions for continuing professional education.

To help bridge the gap separating acupuncturists from MDs, most United States acupuncture schools train students to be familiar with conventional Western medical language. It would serve the interest of patients if this cooperative impulse prevailed in medical schools. One woman, allergic to standard drugs and in her second pregnancy, was delighted when her obstetrician agreed to work with an acupuncturist during delivery. She had some anxious days while the obstetrician sought permission for this patient-oriented team to go into action at the hospital where he was on staff. The hospital refused. In this case, another local hospital agreed to the plan.

The 1980s has seen isolated acupuncturists form local groups; and the birth of an effective national coalition, leading to establishment of acupuncture as an independent profession.

The American Association of Acupuncture and Oriental Medicine (AAAOM) was formed in 1981 to strenghten and promote the profession in orderly fashion. Membership includes acupuncturists, patients, MDs and other people with an interest in acupuncture. Professional members represent numerous acupuncture traditions feeding the development of American acupuncture.

In 1982 a consortium of 11 schools established the National Council of Acupuncture Schools and Colleges (NCASC), "to advance the status of acupuncture and Oriental medicine in the United States." The NCASC considers a 2-year residential program to be the minimum study necessary for certification as an acupuncturist.

The National Commission for the Certification of Acupuncturists (NCCA), sponsored by the AAAOM, became autonomous in 1983. The NCCA has developed accreditation formulas for the older generation of acupuncturists; and designed a standard test to be used in licensing recent and future graduates of acupuncture schools. Professional tests are expensive to design and administer. Many state legislatures see no reason to appropriate money for such testing. The NCCA has produced a standard test of acupuncture competence which states may use as a basis for licensure, without spending money to design their own. Existence of this test should help overcome legislative and regulatory obstacles which result in depriving patients of health-care choices.

Acupuncture advocates have sponsored legislative bills to establish state acupuncture boards. The New Jersey legislature passed such a bill in 1983; and in 1985 was the first state to give the NCCA test. In 1986, Massachusetts passed a similar bill.

At the federal level 2 bills in Congress would make acupuncture coverable by Medicare and Medicaid. Of importance to these bills is another, which proposes removal of the "experimental" label from acupuncture needles.

*   *   *

In the 1840s "regular" medical practitioners in the United States were a somewhat disheveled lot, in sad decline from the elevated social status doctors enjoyed in Colonial times. In post-Jacksonian America, most medical schools were diploma mills. Conventional medicine was not very effective against disease. Doctors were losing patients to "irregular" healers—practitioners of many different kinds of treatment who had one thing in common: their methods were not based on a body of scientific theory, but on observation and experience. Practitioners of scientific medicine as taught in European medical schools and in the few reputable American ones, determined to organize. They would regulate themselves by mutually agreed-upon standards, for the benefit of patients and for their own advancement as career medical people. Clearly there is pattern of similarity between organization of the AMA in 1846; and formation of the AAAOM 135 years later.

*   *   *

The way states view acupuncture practice falls into three broad categories. Some states license acupuncturists and allow them to practice more or less independently; some states do not license them, but unofficially tolerate the practice of acupuncture; and in some states acupuncture may be performed only by an MD, or other Medical Act licensee. Not all states have laws written specifically about acupuncture; among those which do, laws are inconsistent from state to state. Acupuncture regulation is in a slow process of change as states move toward authorizing licensed independent practice.

Current policy about *what* acupuncture is, and *who* may

practice it varies widely. Variations in state policy affect not only your search for treatment, but also your health insurance coverage. Legally-required office procedures, especially those defining acupuncture as "experimental treatment" may have a chilling effect on your intention to try acupuncture. States differ also about the educational requirements for being "fully licensed under the Medical Act." In New York, only dentists and physicians qualify. Other states put chiropractors, osteopaths and podiatrists in this category. In Illinois over 300 chiropractors and podiatrists have taken acupuncture training.

Some states require Medical Act licensees who want to practice acupuncture to take a training course, and/or pass a test. Others don't. In states where an acupuncture training course is required for medical act licensees to give this treatment, study consists at most of 300 hours of lectures, observation and practice. However, some states which license acupuncturists—professionals whose method of health care is limited to acupuncture and Oriental medicine—require proof of 2 or more years of acupuncture education and at least 10 years' practice. This policy reflects an official view that if you've spent years becoming an MD, acupuncture is simply another modality, an additional treatment tool. It is a view with which most acupuncture professionals disagree.

State requirements for medical supervision of acupuncturists vary. Critics of the idea of medical supervision have asked what the requirement really means, when supervising doctors generally have had only limited contact with acupuncture. States define supervision in different degrees of strictness. It can be close personal supervision of someone employed by the doctor's practice to do acupuncture; written referral of the patient to an outside acupuncturist after physical diagnosis by the referring physician; or, least strict in this category, verifiable but informal supervision of an acupuncture practice by a Medical Act licensee. The stricter forms of this type of regulation mean that you must pay for one or more doctor's appointments before beginning acupuncture treatment. In localities with the least strict medical supervision—among them, the District of Columbia, Maryland, Pennsylvania and Utah—you may choose acupuncture directly, without a note from your doctor.

Why are the state regulations haphazard and inconsistent?

Twenty years ago acupuncture was rarely available in the United States outside cities with large Chinese communities. There was no question of licensing, because state governments took the position that Oriental medicine—acupuncture, herbs and massage—was just another aspect of Chinese community cultural affairs, and therefore of no concern to mainstream society.

Starting in 1971, the general public began to show an interest in acupuncture. When demand for treatment was noted outside Chinese communities, acupuncture attracted official attention. At the federal level, the Food and Drug Administration (FDA) labelled acupuncture needles "experimental devices." (To call the acupuncture needle "experimental" is like calling Chinese, Dutch, French or Japanese "experimental" languages, when the label properly applies to the non-native, inexpert speaker, not to the language itself.)

In 1972, the District of Columbia was the first United States jurisdiction to establish acupuncture policy, allowing non-physician acupuncturists to work under direct medical supervision. This same year, when some state governments began to regulate acupuncture practice, they set policy in a hurry, without time for real investigation. Decisions were often based on politics, not on expertise. Many stopgap acupuncture laws have remained unchanged since 1975.

The present confused nature of acupuncture laws tells you nothing about acupuncture. It does show how complicated and difficult it is to integrate an unusual medicine of foreign origin into our health-care establishment. The practical consequences are that you may have to proceed indirectly in your search for an acupuncturist. It's not always a simple matter of flipping through the 'A' section of the telephone directory Yellow Pages, making a list of acupuncturists, and checking them out.

New York and states with similar acupuncture regulation accept foreign credentials only from localities which regulate the practice of acupuncture. Because Hong Kong has no such regulation, experienced acupuncturists who have trained and worked only in Hong Kong are not licensed by the state of New York.

A certain amount of unregulated acupuncture is still practiced in the United States. One acupuncturist displays on his office wall documents which include 6 years as an army physician in his Asian country. He is experienced, but not acceptably so by the standards of the state in which he conducts a busy, if un-licensed, practice. For good professional reasons, an experienced acupuncturist may consider it foolish and degrading to work under direction of someone who knows little about acupuncture. Others feel it is hypocritical, if not unethical, to join forces with an MD for the sole purpose of having the doctor satisfy state policy which is basically anti-acupuncture. Most trained, experienced acupuncturists feel bound to respect their profession by scrupulous regard for the patient's well-being. Generally they see indepen-dent practice, in a well-regulated profession, as the proper framework in which to function.

In a reasonably law-abiding society we assume that professional licensing is a good thing which works for the protec-tion of consumers. As a general rule it is, and does. But a resident of a state which limits the practice of acupuncture to doctors may discover there are no doctors practicing acupuncture; or that a doctor who knows a little acupuncture is not really a qualified acupuncturist; or that a good MD-acupuncturist lives so far away that travel makes treatment virtually impossible.

In 1980 a group of Texas acupuncture patients, in a class action lawsuit, said in court that state law unjustly deprived them of the right to seek acupuncture treatment. Only doctors were allowed to practice acupuncture in Texas; but patients could not get the names of doctors providing this treatment. The group of patients didn't spring up overnight like mushrooms. Despite state policy they had managed to find acupuncture treatment; and valued the therapy enough to get together and attack the rule,

90

which was ultimately declared unconstitutional. In February, 1984, an opinion by the State Attorney General confirmed the unconstitutionality of Texas acupuncture law. In late 1986, acupuncture in Texas is tolerated, but not licensed. Some 12 other states which officially limit the practice of acupuncture to doctors openly tolerate practice by non-MD acupuncturists, who generally have gone to another state for a license or certification. This tolerance means a substantial number of people want acupuncture and have access to practitioners. It is also an indication that changes in state policy may be in the offing.

How do acupuncturists and patients manage in states which actively discourage the profession? What does "underground" practice mean to your search for acupuncture treatment? Patients refer other patients, thus forming a support network for each other, and a relationship of mutual trust with the practitioner. One acupuncturist, certified in Europe, practices in a New England state which views acupuncture as the practice of medicine, and does not license acupuncturists. Her reputation is good enough for local hospitals to refer patients to her. Even when they do not exert pressure for regulatory change, patient-networks make a difference to the acceptability of acupuncture.

Unfortunately, existence of acupuncture as a marginal profession in some states means that the less competent practice along with better, more experienced acupuncturists. This is one reason why advocacy groups urge national standards of proficiency, as well as more sensible legislation.

In acupuncture as in accounting, automotive mechanics or law, certified does not necessarily mean qualified. A competent, reliable acupuncturist will have a good patient-network. The existence of such networks in states which refuse to license non-physician acupuncturists is a pretty good indication that the market will protect you. Inform yourself as thoroughly as possible by talking to patients; check out documents displayed on the office wall; then use your own judgement.

✳   ✳   ✳

Answers to the question, does health insurance cover acupuncture, are: yes, no, sometimes. It depends on the diagnosis, on where you live, on who signs the recommendation for treatment, on who performs the treatment, on the kind of policy you have—the same company can have different guidelines, according to the type of policy—and even on the attitude of the individual claims adjuster. Variables affect each other; and collectively determine your chances of being covered for this type of health care. Private-sector insurance companies in effect have semi-governmental power in setting health-care policy. They can exclude benefits for treatment which the insured person wants, but which is deemed unconventional. Insurance companies also control health care by determining on a satistical basis how many treatments are indicated for a particular condition.

Insurance companies are more likely to pay on acupuncture treatment for pain, than for acupuncture used preventively, or for systemic problems. However, the group health plan of one major corporation covers 75% of costs of acupuncture treatment for employees who want to quit smoking.

Health insurance plans routinely require that acupuncture be recommended by a "primary care provider." One company lists "primary care providers" whose referral makes acupuncture treatment acceptable for coverage, when these professionals are licensed by the proper state authority. In addition to MDs, the list includes Dr. of Osteopathy; Dentist; Dental Surgeon; Dr. of Surgical Chiropody; Dr. of Podiatry; Physician's Assistant; Certified Nurse Practitioner; Psychologist; and Certified Nurse Midwife. State regulations supersede details of a contract. As a general rule, in most states you have a better chance of reimbursement if a doctor refers you to acupuncture.

To a certain extent insurance company definitions of health-care providers reflect state health-professional licensing policies. In California, acupuncture is customary and usual treatment. Under the group health insurance of Screen Actors' Guild (SAG), a member living in California may have treatment from a Certified Acupuncturist (California designation) without prior

MD referral. Up to 40 treatments are coverable at 80% with the standard $200 deduction. Only if the patient needs further treatment is coverage subject to medical review. In New York acupuncture is considered unusual treatment. If a SAG member living in New York files a claim for *any* acupuncture treatment, it is coverable only if accompanied by a doctor's letter referring the person for acupuncture.

Health insurance company regulations are not consistent with each other. While many companies are satisfied by an MD referral to a licensed acupuncturist, one major carrier covers acupuncture only if treatment is *performed* by an MD, as well as *recommended* by one, even though the state in question licenses acupuncturists.

A health insurance company may offer a variety of plans, with different kinds of benefits. Depending on the plan, acupuncture may or may not be covered.

If a large organization shopping for group health insurance wants acupuncture treatment to be coverable, it will be written into the premium. As a substantial customer, the company or union has some say in designing the insurance plan. Individuals also have some power to influence coverage under the group plan to which they subscribe. When employees or union members made it known that they had received effective acupuncture treatment, it has happened that the next time the company or union put out bids for health insurance, it required inclusion of acupuncture as a covered benefit.

The attitude of the claims adjuster may affect acceptance of your claim. Sometimes a subscriber to a group health plan has submitted a claim for acupuncture and been reimbursed, even when acupuncture was not listed as a covered benefit. As far as the insurance company is concerned, the amount of money in such cases is modest; requests for paying on acupuncture come up infrequently; and the insurance company, having sold a substantial group contract, simply goes along with the request.

As a subscriber to group health insurance you were sent a booklet of information about the contract. The booklet may or may not give precise details about coverage of unconventional health care. Your employer, or union, has a copy of the *master contract*. To learn if acupuncture is covered, call the personnel office, or the union's insurance department, and ask for a reading of the relevant section of the master contract.

If you have individual health insurance, submit a claim as soon as you've paid for a few acupuncture treatments. Acupuncture is modestly priced by the standards of conventional medicine, but with a series of treatments, fees mount up.

An Equitable representative said, "We do pay on acupuncture, but an individual must have a policy and submit a claim for treatment. Then we send you guidelines." The company would not mail these guidelines just to satisfy the curiosity of an insurance-shopper. To receive a copy, you must be an insured person submitting a claim after having had treatment.

A Prudential representative in New York City said, "Almost everybody pays on acupuncture." When told that some companies don't, she said, "I write for about ten companies and they all do, so long as it's an acupuncturist licensed by the state of New York."

When you bought individual health insurance you may not have questioned the exclusions. But if insurance coverage makes the difference between having acupuncture, or limiting yourself to conventional treatment, you might want to change your brand of health insurance.

Medicare does not cover acupuncture.

As a rule, Medicaid does not cover acupuncture; but exceptions are made for some patients of some City hospitals.

RESOURCES

Nationwide   American Association of Acupuncture
and Oriental Medicine
50 Maple Place, Manhasset, NY 11030

Center for Chinese Medicine
5266 East Pomona Boulevard
Los Angeles, California 90022

Traditional Acupuncture Institute
American City Building
Columbia, Maryland, 21044
The above organizations have nationwide membership. You may write asking for names of acupuncturists in your
area. Enclose a stamped, self-addressed
envelope. NOTE: these are lists only;
and do not imply recommendation by
the organization.

**State
Associations**

These local societies are organizational
members of AAAOM

Acupuncture and Moxibustion
Association of New Jersey
668 Raritan Road, Clark, NJ 07066

Acupuncture Association of Colorado
1544 Lafayette Street
Denver, CO 80218

Acupuncture Association of Hawaii
1185 Bethel Street, Honolulu, HI 96813

Acupuncture Association of
Metropolitan Washington
4400 East-West Highway
Bethesda, Maryland 20814

Acupuncture Association of Minnesota
P.O. Box 8858, Minneapolis, MN 55408

Acupuncture Medicine Association of
Southern California
P.O. Box 7406, Alhambra, CA 91802

Florida State Acupuncture Association
456 Avenida del Mayo
Sarasota, FL 34242

Illinois State Acupuncture
Association, Inc.
1222 W. Grace, Chicago, IL 60613

Maine Association for Acupuncture and
Oriental Medicine
Box 226, Blue Hill, ME 04614

Maryland Acupuncture Society
1109 Spring Street, Suite 604
Silver Spring, MD 20910

Massachusetts Acupuncture
Society, Inc.
P.O. Box 440
South Framingham, MA 01701

Oregon Acupuncture Association
P.O. Box 14936, Portland, OR 97214

Pennsylvania Acupuncture Association
Alden Park Manor #604B
Philadelphia, PA 19144

The Acupuncture Association of Texas
4119 Montrose Blvd. Suite 112
Houston, TX 77006

Vermont Association of Acupuncture
and Oriental Medicine
204 Pearl St., Burlington, VT 05401

Other Sources of Local Information

Arizona Acupuncture Association
1735 East Fort Lowell, Suite 12
Tucson, Arizona 85719

Acupuncture Society of America
4140 Broadway, Kansas City,
Missouri 40855
In requesting referral, they ask you to
mention this book

Department of Business Regulation
Professional Licensing Division
Heber M. Wells Building
160 East 300 South
P.O. Box 5802
Salt Lake City, Utah 84110
Has statewide listing of acupuncturists

Miscellaneous Resources

Telephone Directory-Consumer Yellow Pages
Although useful, this is seldom a complete listing: some practitioners disapprove of the principle of advertising health care. Other practitioners register with an acupuncture referral service. Different Yellow Pages listings under which you may find acupuncture are Chiropractors, Osteopaths and Podiatrists. In a state which allows acupuncturists to practice only as Physicians Assistants under direct medical

supervision, they do not advertise independently.

East-West in the name of a bookstore, health- or fitness-center, or health-food store means that the business specializes in connecting Asian and Western cultures. You may pick up a lead to an acupuncturist at one of these places.

Holistic (often spelled Wholistic) Health Center: the name implies emphasis on alternative-medicine techniques; therapies usually include acupuncture.

Pain Clinics Chronic-Pain clinics have been established at many medical centers in response to the dreary scenario of the patient who is seen again and again with the same unrelieved pain. The pain clinic approach to chronic problems is multi-modal: if it does no harm, and is known to be effective, an unconventional technique is tried. Acupuncture is often available. The acupuncturist may be on staff; the clinic may refer you to an outside acupuncturist; or such referral may be made only at your request.

Insurance

Consumers United Insurance Company
2100 M Street, NW
Washington, DC 20037
(202) 872-5390; 1-800-424-9711
Literature emphasizes coverage of alternative health-care treatments.

Workmen's Circle, 45 East 33rd Street
New York, NY 10016
(212) 889-6800
Membership in this nationwide organization is $12 quarterly. Group health plan available in some states. Acupuncture is covered in New York. For other states, check local branch.

The following have a record of paying on acupuncture treatment:

Aetna Life & Casualty

Bankers Life Insurance Company of
   Des Moines

Connecticut General Life

Equitable Life Assurance Society

Fireman's Fund Insurance Companies

Hartford Insurance Group

John Hancock Mutual Life Insurance

Liberty Mutual Insurance Companies

Metropolitan Life Insurance

Prudential Insurance Co. of America

Travelers Insurance Companies

SEVEN

Veterinary use of Acupuncture

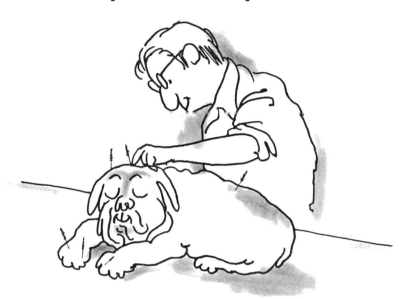

ACUPUNCTURE is a complete medical system which can be used to treat animals as well as humans. In China acupuncture was used in veterinary medicine in the first millenium B.C. At least nine books on the subject had been written by 1000 A.D. The practice of veterinary acupuncture was certainly well established before it was codified in books. A typical title, *Ma Niu I Fang—Veterinary Prescriptions for Horses and Oxen*—printed in 1399, indicates the focus of practice.

Because of their usefulness in battle, trade, and travel, horses were the first animals treated with acupuncture. Dogs as well as horses were treated with veterinary acupuncture in the 7th through 10th centuries A.D.

During the 300 years of sporadic Western interest in acupuncture since the 17th century, some European veterinarians from time to time used acupuncture on horses and cows. In Germany, in the early 19th century, there was a new wave of interest in acupuncture. A number of Viennese veterinary surgeons used it. The mid-century focus on major developments in Western scientific medicine caused this flurry of acupuncture activity to subside, although interest in the subject never completely died out.

In France, the long colonial involvement with Indochina stimulated a current of interest in Chinese medicine which survived the mid-19th century spurt in growth of Western science.

After World War II, there was a revival of veterinary acupuncture in Europe, used mostly on farm animals. Some investigation of veterinary acupuncture was being done in the United States in the 1960s.

In clinical trials of human acupuncture, patients are commonly asked to keep a record of such *objective* data as distance walked each day, amount of medication taken, or hours of uninterrupted sleep. Medical investigators use this information to balance or amplify the patient's own account of response to treatment— the *subjective* report.

Animal behavior reveals health or sickness. Animals don't anticipate the results of treatment; they respond, or fail to respond, without preconception. In judging effectiveness of veterinary acupuncture treatment, objective evidence is all you have. Can the Great Dane resume going up and down stairs, to be taken out for her walks? Is the cat eating? Has fur grown back on bald spots caused by contact dermatitis? Have the lesions of lick granuloma healed? Does the horse no longer favor the left front leg? Is the stallion with the sore back now able to stand at stud? Has the cow, or the pig, become routinely fertile?

Whether or not animals share your life, results of animal treatment challenge the skeptic who says, "Acupuncture works if the problem is in your head. It doesn't work if the problem is real."

* * *

Veterinary practice falls into three main categories: large-animal, small-animal, and exotics.

Veterinarians with a fulltime practice in exotics work in

zoos or animal preserves which retain staff veterinarians.

Large-animal practice concerns the treatment of horses and livestock. Patients come in various sizes, ranging from Percherons to piglets. With few exceptions, patients seen in large-animal practice exist because their owners make a living from them. Illness or incapacity in these animals can destroy a business. In the United States most large-animal veterinary acupuncture is performed on racehorses. However, there are other applications with demonstrated value for commercial livestock. Most of the contemporary reports come from abroad; but some work has been done in this country.

Cows used in commercial diary herds have been selected and bred for generations to produce large amounts of milk. But a heifer—a maiden cow—must produce a calf in order to give milk. Dairy cows are working mothers. A heifer who fails to become pregnant after 4 or 5 inseminations is a dud, and not worth her keep. To prevent total loss on the dairy farmer's investment, such heifers are normally sold for meat. In 1983, the International Veterinary Acupuncture Society (IVAS) newsletter carried a report by a Wisconsin veterinarian that 80% of such dud heifers treated by acupuncture became pregnant after the next insemination. Inexpensive short-term treatment resulted in long-term benefits to owners.

Similar effective use of acupuncture in pigs which had produced unhealthy piglets, or which had failed to come into heat normally after giving birth, has been documented in Taiwan. Successful treatment of delayed puberty in gilts—immature sows—and of sows producing no milk, or milk inadequate to the needs of their offspring, has also been reported. Pigs have also been successfully treated with acupuncture for heatstroke, fevers and diarrhea. Acupuncture leaves no residual substances in these food animals.

Most horses work for a living. Like human athletes and dancers, they are subject to occupational injuries. But with fewer career-change options than humans, horses who can no longer do the work for which they're trained have short futures.

The large mass of a horse's body moves with speed and precision on legs whose lower structure is an intricate assembly of tendons, cartilage and bones of different sizes. The hoof, which from a distance looks like a solid lump of bone, is really quite a vulnerable structure of horny cartilage, flesh, and bone slung in tendons. A problem in any one of these parts affects balance and mobility.

Lower-leg tendons are surrounded and supported by a snug spiral of cartilage. Overexertion can cause gaps in this supportive spiral; with the result that tendons bulge out between the cartilage—a condition known as *bowed tendons*. The navicular, a bone in the hoof, can shift out of place and press against deep tendons, causing pain which drastically interferes with the animal's proper gait. This is called *navicular disease*. *Founder* is a hoof problem of poor blood circulation to the inner rim of the hoof. Horses used for hunting and in shows can develop *back problems* from too much jumping. Aside from musculo-skeletal problems, horses are subject to systemic troubles which don't occur in humans. *Colic*—abdominal pain which can result in torsion, or twisting of the intestines—is agonizing and can be fatal. *Tying up* is similar to colic, but the prevailing sign is muscle spasm.

Bowed tendons, chronic back problems, navicular disease, founder and colic are some of the equine health problems which are being effectively treated by veterinarians using acupuncture. Methods used include classical acupuncture; injection of medication at acupuncture points; electro-acupuncture; and cold laser treatment at acupuncture points. There are other techniques—one racetrack veterinarian is known for using only ear-acupuncture on his patients.

Racehorses are a special category of equine patients in that state regulations dicate when and under what circumstances they may be treated. For example, the California Horse Racing Board specifies that acupuncture or acupunture-related treatment may be given by a licensed veterinarian; or by an acupuncture technician under direct visual supervision of a veterinarian, who must enter the fact of treatment in a book. Except for proven 'bleeders'—horses which bleed from their lungs in a strenuous race, and who may be treated with Lasix (furosemide) before they run—all sports medicine treatment, including acupuncture, is prohibited the day before a race.

Acupuncture is not a quick fix. The veterinarian who treats a horse with acupuncture generally recommends that the patient take it easy for a while, to let the healing effects of acupuncture become well established before the animal resumes work. But when horses are in the racing business, owners and trainers can be impatient, run the horse too soon, then complain about recurrence of the problem.

* * *

Small-animal practice is the care of pets—mostly cats and dogs; they may range in size and shape from Newfoundland to Siamese kitten, but the "small-animal" label still applies. Most veterinary doctors specialize in either large- or small-animal practice; although some rural veterinarians work in both specialities.

The Animal Medical Center (AMC), in New York City, is a hospital where veterinary doctors practice cardiology, neurology, surgery and other conventional medical specialities. In one respect, choice of treatment here is wider than in most United States hospitals for humans. Acupuncture treatment has been available at the AMC since 1982 when Dr. Allen M. Schoen, a graduate of New York State College of Veterinary Medicine, Cornell University, became an AMC consultant.

Dr. Schoen began using acupuncture in his private practice in 1981. He is a Board member of the International Veterinary Acupuncture Society (IVAS). IVAS has been training United States veterinarians in acupuncture since 1974.

When he became associated with the AMC, Dr. Schoen began commuting weekly from his practice in Westchester County, N.Y. Acupuncture was new to the AMC, a prestigious veterinary setting. It took time to demonstrate its value; and to overcome skepticism on the part of some staff members. For the first year, he would drive an hour and a half into the city to treat one patient, then turn around and drive back. After a discouragingly slow period, things changed.

In the fall of 1984, he was keeping two treatment rooms busy with animals referred for acupuncture. In the summer of 1985, he was assisted by Dr. Rick Joseph, an AMC veterinary intern, who was taking the IVAS acupuncture course. By this time Dr. Schoen's patients kept three treatment rooms busy during his weekly visits. In the spring of 1986, Dr. Joseph—now an AMC resident in neurology—received his IVAS certificate. With Dr. Schoen still acting as Dr. Joseph's preceptor, a second night could now be scheduled for Dr. Joseph to see those patients for whom twice-weekly treatment was desirable.

With animals, as with people, it is often more effective to give acupuncture twice a week in the initial stages of treating a problem; then, as the acupuncture effect takes hold, to stretch out intervals between treatments. For therapeutic reasons, Dr. Schoen had wanted the second weekly session from the beginning. With increased demand for acupuncture by AMC clients, and Dr. Joseph's certification, it was now practical to expand the schedule.

As one client said, "The once a week schedule was really because that's the only time the doctor was available—twice a week would have been better."

Patients are brought to Dr. Schoen's Westchester County practice for both conventional and acupuncture treatment. At the AMC, where he is the acupuncture specialist, patients are referred for acupuncture treatment. These referrals come from the AMC Emergency Room; from other veterinarians, either AMC staff members or in private practice; and from clients whose animals have been helped by acupuncture.

Dr. Schoen is a dark-haired, bearded man in his mid-thirties who listens intently to clients while assessing their pets, his patients. Despite appointments scheduled at fifteen-minute intervals, he gives the impression of having endless time available for each case.

A man brings in a dachshund, which has had surgery—laminectomy—for a back problem. The condition was not cured, and the dog is on cortisone; the owner is unsure if this is meant to be long-term or short-term treatment. His regular veterinarian referred him to consult about acupuncture, which the owner hopes will be better for the dog than continuing cortisone treatment.

"I stopped the cortisone last night," the man says.

Dr. Schoen observes the dog. He says he can't evaluate—the dog seems fine, but may still have cortisone in his system. (If so, this medication is still preventing development of inflammation; so there's no way to know if the condition which triggers inflammation is still present.)

"It doesn't make sense to treat him with acupuncture right now."

The man seems eager to have the dog treated.

"If the condition recurs, we'll try acupuncture," says Dr. Schoen.

The man looks relieved.

Dr. Schoen is a strong advocate for appropriate use of acupuncture; but like any responsible practitioner, is no fanatic. When he believes that he cannot help a particular client with acupuncture, or when circumstances make acupuncture unsuitable, he doesn't hesitate to say so. Like humans, animals in the United States often receive acupuncture treatment after various conventional remedies have failed to improve a condition. Even in these last-resort cases, satisfactory results have been documented: physiological function has been improved or restored, with resulting improvement in quality of the animal's life.

Thomas is a 9½ year old pug. One day, walking on the beach, his owner noticed trailing claw marks on the dog's track in the sand. Soon Thomas showed signs of weakness in his hind legs. X-ray revealed calcium deposits on vertebrae, in places that would make surgery very risky. Because of the poor chances for successful surgery, his owner decided to try acupuncture.

This treatment session was observed in July, 1984, when Thomas had been receiving acupuncture for several months; and was on a maintenance regime of treatment every two weeks. However, because the people involved had scheduling conflicts, the latest interval was three weeks.

"It was too long," says his owner, as Thomas walks slowly into the treatment room, and sits in the corner. He shows none of the usual canine interest in exploring the area; and yelps twice when lifted to the treatment table. His owner sits at the end of the table, facing the dog, holding him lightly. Thomas lies on his stomach. He does not try to leave the table, as dogs often do when they have felt pain during a routine procedure.

His owner remarks that Thomas regularly objected to the insertion of two particular needles. Now, he shields Thomas's eyes. The needles go into the dog's front paws, with no objection from Thomas. In a few minutes, his nose becomes damp—a standard reaction to stimulus from the front-paw needles. Dr. Schoen places more needles in two lines parallel to Thomas's cervical and thoracic vertebrae. Thomas yawns. He appears completely unaware of the needles going in.

Treatment continues. Two needles in the cervical region are attached by clips to a battery-driven electro-pulsator. Despite the visible twitching this causes, and with nineteen needles in place, the dog's lids droop over his prominent pug eyes. Thomas dozes.

About twenty minutes later the needles are removed. Thomas is lifted down to the floor. He shakes himself as if coming out of water, then romps around the room, wagging his tail so energetically that his whole rear end wiggles.

In dogs, yawning, tail-wagging and jumping around are behavioral signs of pleasure. Thomas moves freely and normally; the physiological improvement is evident. According to his owner, this improvement persists during the regular intervals between maintenance treatments; but there is some relapse if the interval is extended. Samantha, the 12-year-old mother of Thomas, is also in treatment, for arthritic shoulders.

In November, 1985, sixteen months later, these dogs were again observed at a treatment session.

Talking while he puts needles into Thomas, who pays no attention, Dr. Schoen asks the owner if treatment is helping *his* condition. The man smiles and explains.

"It might interest you," he says, "to know that I've begun to get acupuncture treatment for my sinus." He names his practitioner, a well-respected Taiwan-born acupuncturist and teacher. "Usually it starts with the first cold damp weather, and lasts until I can go somewhere warm, no matter what I do. The acupuncture is the only treatment that's helped me."

He and Dr. Schoen talk about the fact that Thomas and Samantha have shown no deterioration of their respective conditions, which normally get worse with time. However, for these dogs it has not been possible to stretch the treatment intervals beyond 2 weeks.

At rates charged by the AMC, the owner is spending $1,300 for a year of treatment. A well-informed, solicitous and observant man, he is willing to commit time and money to keep Thomas and Samantha in a state of well-being.

"I'm convinced it's because of acupuncture that these two are still in my life," he says.

✳ ✳ ✳

In response to inquiries about veterinary acupuncture, a staff member at a lower Manhattan veterinary clinic said, "Nobody here does it, but one of our clients has had good luck with it."

Harold agreed to an interview at his place of business, in company with Vibrato, a Toy Fox Terrier.

"He had a stroke when he was 15," says Harold, looking over from his desk at Vibrato, curled up nearby in a flattened green bag. "His regular vet said, since it was an old dog, nothing could be done. But it just happened I was watching the "Today" show, and there was a veterinarian acupuncturing a dog, so I called him up."

"What's his name?"

"Dr. Allen Schoen. I took Vibrato up to his clinic in Westchester County. He had the stroke in March, and this was in September."

In dogs, paralysis lasting 4 months is normally deemed

paralysis for life. When taken for his first acupuncture treatment 6 months after the stroke, says Harold, "Vibrato presented with some muscle atrophy and arthritis. He absolutely could not walk at all. Dr. Schoen said he was the smallest animal he'd ever treated.

"He put needles in his back, hind legs and knees. At first Vibrato squealed—" each time his name is spoken, the dog picks up his head and stares brightly at Harold, then drops his nose to his paws when nothing further attracts his attention.

"—then after a few minutes the endorphins started, and he became lethargic, and his heartbeat slowed. Some of the needles were electrically stimulated.

"Dr. Schoen also gave some nutritional advice—stop feeding him my leftover cereal and milk. And we changed to a different canned food. It took three days to switch him over, but I managed, I'd give him a treat and some vitamins, just to make sure he got the nutrition."

Initially Vibrato had 8 or 10 treatments; after that, booster treatments every three or four weeks.

"Later, we went to the Animal Medical Center—Dr. Schoen works there once a week. After treatment Vibrato is very lethargic, he rides in that shoulder bag back to Queens on the subway from the East Side. Then he wants to eat. His appetite has really increased since he started treatment."

Harold picks Vibrato up, and strokes him.

"Don't try to pat him while I'm holding him—he may be small, but he's very protective."

He sets the dog—the size of an average cat—on the floor, where Vibrato proceeds to investigate the interviewer. His right hip is somewhat withered; and he does not put weight on the right hind leg. From time to time he curls that paw up, like a bird's claw. But he expresses interest in this stranger crouched on the floor, parading around several times until, curiosity satisfied, he allows himself to be patted.

"He's not at his best today, with this damp cold weather—but neither am I, my sciatica's acting up." As Harold speaks, Vibrato seems to levitate onto his lap, looking confidently up to the man's face. "We've gained a year. He'll be 16 next month."

Harold and his dog appear to thrive on each other's company. Even though his leg is not perfectly normal, Vibrato gets about efficiently, without signs of pain.

❋   ❋   ❋

A woman whose 12 year old English Sheepdog, Robinson, was responding well to acupuncture treatment for arthritic hips and knees, reported that a neighbor said to her, 'I feel so sorry for your dog, I don't know why you don't put him to sleep.'

"I felt like saying maybe the next time *he* had a pain his wife should put *him* to sleep. And it really isn't any of his business."

Observed at his 5th weekly treatment, Robinson stood up easily after lying on the floor. When he first came for treatment, he had to struggle to get to his feet.

Pets are important in our 20th century Western culture: we consider it normal to buy special food for them and to pay for their health care, according to our means. Small animals are big business in this country, as you know from the number of petfood commercials which bombard us on TV. Numerically, pets constitute the majority of veterinary patients. But in the early 1970s United States veterinarians in small-animal practice, who wanted to learn about acupuncture, discovered there were no Chinese acupuncture charts for dogs and cats.

For most of its history, Chinese veterinary treatment, including acupuncture, was limited to animals important for human survival in an agricultural society: horses, camels, cattle, fowl and pigs. Cats and dogs were not economically significant.

Reopening of relations with China in the early 1970s stimulated awareness of Oriental medicine in the United States. Dissatisfied with limitations of conventional treatment, some veterinarians became interested in learning about acupuncture. Many of them started by studying human acupuncture.

Fundamental acupuncture principles are the same for

veterinary and human patients, although details vary. For example, anatomical landmarks by which you locate points differ from species to species; but if you visualize the front legs of your cat or dog as arms, you can see the mammalian similarity. In humans, a major analgesic point is located between the thumb and forefinger. In horses, this point is above each front hoof. In cats and dogs, the anatomical landmark is the dew-claw, analogous to our thumb. Also, in transposing human point location to animals, allowance must be made for the fact that horses have 18 ribs; dogs and cats, 13; and humans, 12. Veterinary applications of acupuncture also vary from the human model. For example, animals have points which don't exist in humans, such as the one at the tip of the tail. However, keeping in mind the differences between species, it was possible to develop small-animal acupuncture charts based on human acupuncture charts.

Studying acupuncture while engaged in conventional veterinary practices, these doctors at first tried their new skill, when owners permitted, on animals slated for euthanasia. Generally such animals suffered the debilitating and degenerative diseases of old age; had been hit by cars; or were wounded in some way. A number of these recent veterinary pioneers have told how they astonished themselves when, practicing what they'd learned in acupuncture class, they had unexpected treatment successes.

For some veterinarians, there were surprising personal benefits. As one said, "When I first was doing acupuncture, I found I was treating myself all the time, using acupressure."

As the body of experience, documented cases, and shared information grew during the 1970s, U.S. veterinarians treated an increasingly wider range of problems with acupuncture and acupuncture-related techniques. In addition to musculo-skeletal problems, other conditions effectively treated in both large- and small-animals include fertility, gastrointestinal, and skin problems. By 1984, according to one expert, about 400 veterinarians in the United States were using acupuncture—learned from various sources—regularly in their practices. IVAS training has been available in this country since 1974. At present

90 IVAS-certified veterinarians practice nationwide, 8 of them in New York State.

Taking your pet for acupuncture treatment does not have to mean signing on for years of veterinary appointments, as the following cases show.

Lucy, an 8 year old spayed lab-retriever cross, twisted her back playing tug-of-war with her owner on an icy sidewalk. Suddenly, she was back-crippled. John, her owner, brought her to the Emergency Room at the AMC. She was examined, and put on a standard course of painkiller medication. John observed that Lucy resumed running and playing, but her condition did not improve, a fact which was obvious if her dosage was delayed. John figured the pills were masking Lucy's pain without contributing to any cure.

Some years ago John had successful acupuncture treatment to quit smoking. Recently, a friend's low-back pain was effectively treated with acupuncture. John wondered if acupuncture could benefit Lucy. He wasn't sure there was such a thing as veterinary acupuncture; but he asked at the AMC and was referred to Dr. Schoen.

Treated by Dr. Schoen, Lucy exhibited a pattern of response familiar to some human patients. Her condition improved visibly after the first and second treatments. After the third, John reported a reversal. However, she showed steady improvement following treatments 5, 6 and 7. John notes that with acupuncture, unlike her behavior while on medication, Lucy's activity is self-regulating according to how she feels. Going to their apartment she will run up one flight of stairs, then walk the next two. With medication she tended to overexert herself.

With John kneeling at her head, Lucy lies calmly on the floor receiving treatment not with the usual needles, or needles and electrostimulation, but with *aquapuncture*. This is a method of stimulating energy by injecting saline solution and vitamin B12 into acupuncture points.

Dr. Schoen and John confer. They agree that Lucy's progress indicates this is her last treatment, barring a new trauma.

Schoen suggests that John continue to observe Lucy, and let the healing which has begun take hold, thus giving her a chance to benefit from the cumulative effects of acupuncture.

"If we'd had to go into surgery," says John, "I would have had her put down. It's the pain, and thousands of dollars."

With a swish of her tawny plumed tail, Lucy hauls him out the door.

* * *

Boston is a beautifully marked black male cat with four white, 6-toed paws. His owners found him on Fire Island, and estimate his age at 10 or 11. (All 6-toed cats trace their ancestry to to Boston, Massachusetts, where the gene-pool for polydactylism originated.) Boston is being treated for allergic dermatitis.

"He sleeps on our bed," says one of his owners, "and you'd hear him licking and licking. I'd wake up and put out my hand to stop him, and he'd lick my hand. All his underpinnings became bald."

Boston had 1½ years of cortisone shots, which the owners were taught to administer. His condition did not improve; and he was referred for acupuncture treatment. He had 2 treatments, 1 week apart. The licking stopped. The third treatment was to be two weeks after the second; but Boston began licking again after 10 days. (This was before the second weekly acupuncture session was instituted at AMC.) The licking stopped again after the third treatment.

Before proceeding to treat Boston, Dr. Schoen holds him up to examine the problem area in bright light. You have to look closely to see the difference between newly-grown black fur, and fur that had not been eroded. The new pelt appears thinner, finer and slightly less glossy than what surrounds it; but the formerly bald skin is completely covered with new growth.

Boston crouches in dignified silence as 2 needles are placed adjacent to his spine and another near the base of his neck. Dr. Schoen tells the owners that, with the good results so far, this fourth treatment will probably be the last.

＊　＊　＊

Appledore is a first-time patient, a substantial female domestic shorthair with tiger markings and white chest. In early youth she was a street cat, scrounging to survive in an alley behind a bar. The man who rescued her from deprived kittenhood ten years ago removes Appledore from her carrying case.

"She's been down on her hocks for about a week," he says. "We brought her to the Emergency Room, but there was no diagnosis."

Determined to regain the security of her carrier, Appledore bellies across the floor. Her left hind paw curls back. (A human with this problem would be walking on the arch, rather than the sole, of the foot.)

Dr. Joseph picks Appledore up and calms her by stroking around the eyes and down her back. Eventually she accepts being set down on the treatment table.

"You better watch from outside," Dr. Schoen says. "I'm treating this cat for the first time, and without any tranquillizer."

Cats tend to be more nervous about acupuncture treatment than dogs.

In the corridor, watching through the window, Appledore's other owner says that she can't stand seeing anyone cut or having injections. She is relieved to hear that the procedure is relatively painfree; and that what pain there is doesn't last. She talks about the aches and pains of aging, and says she thinks acupuncture might be good for her mother; then wonders if it would help her own sciatica.

Appledore appears wary, but lies still, on her stomach, while needles are placed at one-inch intervals in two rows parallel to her spine. Later, as he removes needles, Dr. Schoen is asked how he knows a particular cat will tolerate initiation of treatment. (Needles placed at certain points have a calming effect which takes a few minutes to induce.)

"You have to size them up, you go on intuition." He looks at Appledore, an amiable blob of fur under his hands. "You're just a meatloaf," he tells her.

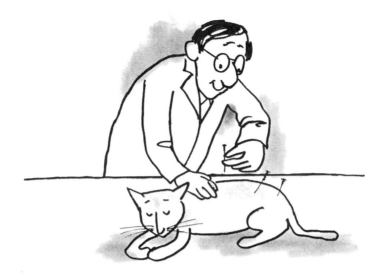

Arriving for her seventh weekly treatment, Appledore is as reluctant to be removed from her carrier as she was six weeks ago. Her owner sets her on the floor, diagonally across the room from the carrying case. She covers ground at all possible speed, her gait watched intently by eight human eyes. The left hind paw no longer curls backward—the release of contraction is well established, her owner says. She is still somewhat down on her hocks, but steps freely; and she stretches her hind leg muscles, instead of favoring them as she crosses the floor.

Appledore is placed on the table. Her owner squats at her head. Dr. Joseph strokes her back a few times. Dr. Schoen places needles parallel to the cat's spine: two rows on the left, one row on the right. Others go into hip, knee and hock. 4 needles are clipped to wires running to the electro-stimulator. The 18 needles are to remain in place for about 5 minutes. After a minute, Appledore clutches the edge of the table with her front claws in a halfhearted attempt to leave this place and get back to her carrier. A few words from her owner, and she curls her paws under her chest. She remains still while needles are removed from her back; but repeats the mildly agitated behavior when the last needles are being withdrawn from her left leg. Her owner puts her into the carrier, where she settles into "meatloaf" pose. Conferring with Appledore's owner Dr. Schoen suggests one more treatment—for a total of 8—and then 2 weeks off. After that, another treatment series may or may not be indicated.

"The nerves appear to be regenerating. We ought to give it a chance to continue by itself."

✽ ✽ ✽

In animals, as in people, it is not always precisely clear at what stage of treatment you've reached the level of maximum benefit. Impatience on the part of practitioners as well as clients can lead to terminating treatment just short of really good results. On the other hand, it is unfair to clients to suggest treatment after treatment without clearly explained reasons and options. An experienced and responsible acupuncturist knows when to stop treatment and allow for the cumulative effect. Acupuncture is art as well as science. As in other arts, less is often more . . .

Buck is tan, with a shepherd tail and stand-up ears that flop over at the tips. Lloyd rescued him from Riverside Park, in New York City, where the dog skulked under an abandoned car. Lloyd believes Buck is 3 or 4 years old—he weighs 54 pounds. Two months before Buck was observed in treatment, he suffered a sudden onset of enormous lumps, bodywide and at the joints.

"He had to tuck the hip-girdle to one side in order to lie down," said Lloyd's wife, Maria. "He was whimpering in pain. He'd cry out, and limp."

Buck was given conventional veterinary treatment: antibiotics and high doses of cortisone. The prognosis was that he'd need cortisone maintenance for the rest of his life. Maria and Lloyd were uneasy about long-term cortisone treatment.

"We know someone who does acupressure," Maria continued, "and she agreed to try treating Buck. The lumps, which were like soft golfballs, decreased. But they didn't go away."

Maria and Lloyd permitted observation of Buck's treatment at a private Manhattan veterinary clinic.

"Wonderful. But we ought to clear it with your vet.

What's his name?"

"Dr. Allen Schoen," said Maria.

Buck lunges into the treatment room as if it were full of steak. It is hard to imagine this lively, cheerful animal has ever been sick. Lloyd says that Buck was back to almost normal activity after 2 treatments. It is now two weeks since the 3rd treatment. Lloyd gets down on the floor with Buck, who wants to play. Dr. Schoen squats, and moves nimbly around treating Buck with aquapuncture—the B12 and saline solution injections—at acupuncture points in his front paws, elbows, upper back and knees.

"Basically, what I'm doing is tonifying the immune system," Dr. Schoen says.

Buck calms down and lies quiet as treatment progresses. He makes no complaint. The minute Dr. Schoen finishes, Buck springs to his feet and wriggles from head to tail. Dr. Schoen and Lloyd discuss Buck's progress and plan future treatments: another—the 5th—in two weeks; the 6th a month after that; and the 7th two months after the 6th.

"Catching it so early, we have a good chance of cure, rather than just treatment," Dr. Schoen says.

The distinction between treatment and cure has special consequences for animal owners. Humans, for the most part, are obliged to live with their maladies. We are equipped to be rational and to adapt to damaged health in extraordinary ways. But in veterinary health care the owner must decide if it is wise or practical to continue treating an animal whose condition recurs when treatment is stopped. In untreatable conditions, you may give your pet the last responsible care: euthanasia. It's tough on you, but less tough on the animal than living miserably or enduring painful death. It has been observed that animals treated with acupuncture tend, when the time comes, to have relatively peaceful natural deaths, not agonizing or convulsive ones.

RESOURCES:

You may request names of veterinarians practicing acupuncture in your region from these organizations. Enclose a stamped, self-addressed envelope or postcard when you write.

> International Veterinary Acupuncture Society
> Meredith Snader, VMD
> Executive Director, IVAS
> R.D. #1, Chester Springs
> Pennsylvania 19425
>
> National Association for Veterinary Acupuncture
> P.O. Box 5181
> Fullerton
> California 92635

APPENDIX I

World Health Organization (WHO) list of provisional list of diseases that lend themselves to acupuncture treatment. List is based on clinical experience, not necessarily on clinical research with controls. The list was formulated at the WHO Interregional Seminar on Acupuncture, Moxibustion and Acupuncture Anesthesia, held in Peking in June, 1979.

UPPER RESPIRATORY TRACT
Acute sinusitis
Acute rhinitis
Common cold
Acute tonsillitis

RESPIRATORY SYSTEM
Acute bronchitis
Bronchial asthma (most effective in children and in
   patients without complicating diseases)

DISORDERS OF THE EYE
Acute conjunctivitis
Central retinitis
Myopia (in children)
Cataract (without complications)

DISORDERS OF THE MOUTH
Toothache, post-extraction pain
Gingivitis
Acute and chronic pharyngitis

GASTRO-INTESTINAL DISORDERS
Spasms of oesophagus and cardia
Hiccough
Gastroptosis
Acute and chronic gastritis
Gastric hyperacidity
Chronic duodenal ulcer (pain relief)
Acute duodenal ulcer (without complications)
Acute and chronic colitis
Acute bacillary dysentery
Constipation
Diarrhoea
Paralytic ileus

NEUROLOGICAL AND MUSCULO-SKELETAL DISORDERS
Headache and migraine
Trigeminal neuralgia
Facial palsy (early stage, i.e., within three to six
    months)
Pareses following a stroke
Peripheral neuropathies
Sequelae of poliomyelitis (early stage, i.e., within
    six months)
Meniere's disease
Neurogenic bladder dysfunction
Nocturnal enuresis
Intercostal neuralgia
Cervicobrachial syndrome
"Frozen shoulder," "tennis elbow"
Sciatica
Low back pain
Osteoarthritis

APPENDIX II

I received 98 replies to a newspaper notice asking to hear from people who had had acupuncture treatment. 19 were not fully responsive, so do not apply. This informal, unscientific analysis is, therefore, based on 79 anecdotal reports. Of these, 80% reported positive results.

16 people reported ineffective treatment: some had no response; some had strongly adverse comments on practitioners; some reported only fleeting relief of problem.

4 people reported fairly beneficial treatment: acupuncture worked pretty well, but not well enough to motivate continued or repeated treatment.

15 people reported satisfactory treatment: they have had good results; and continue to get acupuncture treatment for preventive maintenance at intervals ranging from monthly to semi-annually.

44 people reported good results of acupuncture treatment: they were enthusiastic; often surprised because they had expected little benefit; and described substantial longterm relief with no recurrence of the health problem since last treatment—as much as 10 years ago.

Age Range: 50 people gave the age at which they first tried acupuncture. Willingness to try unfamiliar therapy was not limited to young people: 35 of these patients were over 40 when first treated.

BIBLIOGRAPHY

Barefoot Doctor's Manual: The American Translation of the Chinese Paramedical Manual — Running Press, Philadelphia, 1977

Acupuncture — Felix Mann, M.B. Vintage Books, New York 1973

Acupuncture, A Comprehensive Text — John O'Connor & Dan Bensky, translators & editors Shanghai College of Traditional Medicine. Eastland Press, Chicago, 1981

Acupuncture for Americans — Louise Oftedal Wensel, M.D. Reston Publishing Company, 1980

Acupuncture for Patients — Teruo Matsumoto, M.D. Charles C. Thomas, Illinois, 1975

Acupuncture Manual, A Western Approach — Luke S.W. Chu, M.D., *et alia,* Marcel Dekker, Inc., New York, 1979

Acupuncture Medicine	Yoshiaki Omura, Sc.D.,M.D. Japan Publications, Inc., Tokyo, 1982
An Introduction to Acupuncture	Johannes Bischko, M.D. trans. by Diana Reese-Soltesz Karl F. Haug Verlag, Heidelberg, 1978
Celestial Lancets	Lu Gwei-Djen & Joseph Needham Cambridge University Press, Great Britain, 1980
Essentials of Chinese Acupuncture	Foreign Language Press, Beijing, 1980
Fundamentals of Chinese Medicine	Paradigm Publications, Brookline, MA, 1986
Health and Healing	Andrew Weil, M.D. Houghton Mifflin, Boston, 1983
Modern Chinese Acupuncture	Lewith & Lewith Thorsons Publishers Ltd. Great Britain, 1980
The Web That Has No Weaver	Ted J. Kaptchuk Congdon & Weed, New York, 1983
Traditional Medicine and Health Care Coverage	Robert H.O. Bannerman, *et alia*, editors World Health Organization, Geneva, 1983

ORDER FORM

_____ copies of
PLAIN TALK ABOUT ACUPUNCTURE
@ $8.95, plus shipping

	Shipping Charges				
	Within U.S.A.			Outside U.S.A.	
Carrier	U.P.S.	U.P.S. Air	4th Class	Sea Mail	Air Mail
First Book	2.00	6.00	1.25	2.00	18.00
Each Add.	.50	3.00	.60	1.00	7.00

Name:

Street:

City:

State: Zip:

Ship By: UPS ☐   UPS AIR ☐   4th Class ☐   SEA ☐   AIR ☐

Quantity discount price available on request.
All orders take 2-4 weeks for delivery.

Check or money order.
New York residents add appropriate
state/local sales tax.

send to:

Whalehall, Inc.
277 West End Avenue
#15 A
New York, NY 10023

NOTES

Ellinor R. Mitchell is a writer who likes to play classical guitar. She lives in New York City and Chilmark, Massachusetts. Her interest in writing about acupuncture started when treatment relieved finger pains which had made her dread guitar-practice. People said, "You really had acupuncture? Why? What's it like? Did it do any good? How does it work?"

She expected to assemble a list of acupuncture questions-and-answers in a couple of months. But the subject was richer and more complex than she had expected; and totally absorbing. She found herself thinking about acupuncture when she wasn't paying attention to other matters. The list grew into a book.

In nearly 5 years of attending conferences and lectures; and interviewing acupuncture patients and acupuncturists, she has accumulated debts of gratitude, but no obligations; and made no agreement to carry messages.